Meal Prep Cookbook

Plan, Prepare, and Portion Your Whole Food Meals

Table of Contents

Introduction..- 7 -

Benefits of Meal Prep ....- 9 -

Food Prep Containers ....- 12 -

Your Meal Plan and Grocery List...............................- 13 -

Shopping & Storing ....- 16 -

Food Prep...- 18 -

Poultry Recipes..- 19 -

   Chicken Rice & Veggie Bowl ....- 21 -

   Healthy Chicken Fajita with Brown Rice ....- 23 -

   Honey-Lime Chicken with Sweet Potatoes & Asparagus - 25 -

   Chicken Mozzarella Pasta with Tomato Sauce ....- 27 -

   BBQ Chicken Drumsticks and Spaghetti Squash ....- 29 -

   Buffalo Chicken Casserole ....- 31 -

   Chicken Pizza ....- 33 -

   Chicken Enchilada Bowl ....- 34 -

   Pan-roasted Chicken with Couscous and Arugula ....- 36 -

   Garlic Parmesan Chicken Tenders with Green Beans.. - 38 -

   Creamy Garlic Chicken Zucchini Noodles ....- 40 -

   Easy Chicken & Asparagus Sheet Pan ....- 41 -

   Chicken Curry and Couscous ....- 42 -

   Chipotle Shredded Chicken with Cilantro Slaw .... - 44 -

   Chicken Tuscan Pasta Bake .... - 46 -

   Moroccan Chicken with Veggies and Lemon Couscous - 48 -

Roasted Chicken and Veggies with Miso-Honey Butter .- 50 -

Teriyaki Chicken with Rice and Veggies.........................- 52 -

Chicken Shawarma with Sweet Potato Fry....................- 54 -

Greek Chicken with Quinoa and Cucumber Salad ....- 56 -

Easy Jerk Chicken ....- 58 -

Chicken Butternut Squash Pasta ....- 59 -

Italian Chicken Bowls .... - 61 -

Chicken in Peanut Lemon Sauce ....- 63 -

Ground Turkey Taco Bowls ....- 65 -

Thai Basil Ground Turkey...- 67 -

Turkey Burgers & Sweet Potato Fries.......................... - 69 -

Roasted Turkey Breast & Vegetables.............................. - 71 -

Egg Recipes...- 73 -

Scrambled Eggs with Turmeric ....- 75 -

Sausage Hash Brown Casserole ....- 76 -

Veggie Egg Muffins ....- 77 -

Healthy Breakfast Pizza ....- 79 -

Breakfast Stuffed Bell Peppers ....- 81 -

Seafood Recipes ....- 83 -

Roasted Salmon with Vegetables.....................................- 85 -

Salmon Fajita ....- 87 -

Salmon with Bok Choy and Mushrooms ....- 88 -

Salmon with Potatoes and Riced Cauliflower ....- 90 -

Garlic Ginger Basil Salmon...- 91 -

Tuna, Veggie and Quinoa Salad....................................- 93 -

Tuna Poke Bowl ....- 94 -

Creamy Tuna Noodle Casserole.................................- 95 -

Fish Taco Quinoa Bowls ....- 97 -

Sheet Pan Cod with Mushrooms and Onion .... - 99 -

Chinese Style Baked Cod.................................- 100 -

One Pan Baked Cod with Vegetables.................... - 101 -

Sheet Pan Pineapple Shrimp with Bell Peppers..........- 102 -

Shrimp & Chickpea Pasta ....- 103 -

Shrimp, Veggies, and Cauliflower Rice ....- 105 -

Shrimp and Cilantro-Lime Quinoa Bowl...................- 106 -

Halibut with Peach and Pepper Salsa.....................- 108 -

Pan-Fried Trout with Tomato Basil Sauce .... - 110 -

Tilapia in Coconut-Curry Sauce...........................- 111 -

Baked Tilapia with Garlic Breadcrumbs.................... - 113 -

Beef Recipes .... *- 114 -*

Chipotle and Paprika Eye Round Roast .... - 116 -

Beef and Zucchini Noodles Lasagna......................... - 118 -

Steak Bites...- 120 -

Quick and Easy Meatballs................................ - 121 -

Beef Burgers with Vegetables .... - 122 -

One Pot Salsa Beef Skillet ....- 123 -

Bleu Cheese Petit Sirloin...............................- 125 -

One Pot Steak & Potatoes .... - 127 -

Korean Ground Beef and Brown Rice Bowls..............- 128 -

Stuffed Mexican-Style Bell Peppers...........................- 130 -

Pork Recipes ....*- 132 -*

Pork Chop Ranch Sheet Pan .... - 134 -

Herb-Crusted Pork Chops.................................- 136 -

Balsamic Pork Chops with Peppers ....- 138 -

Molasses-Orange Pork Chops with Skillet-Roasted Sweet Potatoes...- 139 -

Pork Cutlets with Beans and Bell Peppers .... - 141 -

Dijon Pork with Fruits and Quinoa ....- 143 -

Ginger Pork Lettuce Wraps ....- 144 -

Pork Tenderloin with Carrots and Potatoes.................- 146 -

Spicy Pulled Pork ....- 147 -

BBQ Pulled Pork Bowls..- 149 -

Creamy Pulled Pork Pasta...- 151 -

Veggie, Lentil & Whole Grain Recipes...........................- 153 -

Lentil Bowl with Feta and Veggies .... - 155 -

Sesame-Ginger Fried Rice .... - 157 -

Simple Tofu Scramble Breakfast .... - 159 -

One Pot Black Bean & Pumpkin Chili........................ - 161 -

Creamy Butternut Squash Pasta with Mushrooms .....- 163 -

Chickpea and Lentil Curry ....- 165 -

Burrito Bowl with Black Beans .... - 167 -

Lentil Salad with Olives and Cucumbers.....................- 168 -

Lentil Shepherd's Pie with Mushrooms and Sweet Potatoes ....- 170 -

Honey-Roasted Brussels Sprouts with Lentil-Quinoa Pilaf.- 172 -

Turkish-Style White Beans Salad ....- 174 -

Lentil Bolognese Pasta..- 176 -

Thai-Style Quinoa Salad with Lime Vinaigrette..........- 178 -

Polenta Bowls with Caramelized Onions and Kale .....- 180 -

Vegetable Enchilada... - 181 -

Orange Ginger Tofu ....- 183 -

Simple Vegetable Fried Rice ....- 185 -

Healthy Ramen Noodle Salad..- 187 -

Baked Sticky Sesame Cauliflower ....- 189 -

Greek-Style Kale Salad with Feta .... - 191 -

Wild Rice with Beets and Pecans...................................- 193 -

Snack and Dessert Recipes ....*- 195 -*

Blueberry Pancake Bites .... - 197 -

Healthy Energy Bars ....- 199 -

Banana Coconut Cookies ....- 200 -

Sweet Energy Bites..- 201 -

Multi-Seed Crackers...- 202 -

Conclusion ....*- 204 -*

Introduction

You don't have to eat less. You just have to eat right!

It's a well-known fact that proper nutrition is a crucial point for our general health. Ideally, we want to eat home cooked whole foods with enough variety to provide us with all needed nutrients. However, who has time to prepare food every day in our busy lives?

Thanks to meal prep, you can eat delicious food and maintain a balanced, healthy diet. Also, you will learn how to save both of your precious things – your time and your money by mastering the food-prepping process. Indeed, having a food prep container filled with your favorite healthy meal saves your minutes and your dollars. Moreover, it eliminates the stress of figuring out what to eat every single time. You don't have to worry about your cravings and going out to eat when you're working. Meal prep makes your healthy living so easy that it fills like a magic!

Don't be afraid to start small; you should build your own meal prep gradually, without getting overwhelmed. Even just prepping lunches or snacks will be a great beginning! What's your schedule look like? At least, you should be eating a breakfast, lunch, and dinner. Obviously, it's all about finding a healthy balance as with everything else in our life.

Never force yourself to eat certain health foods if you don't like them. Instead, choose healthy versions of the foods you like, such as spiralized veggie noodles as an alternative to pasta. Anyway, there is a wide variety of healthy foods to choose from so you definitely can enjoy the health advantages of whole foods without compromising on taste and flavor.

Good carbs found in whole grains, lean proteins, and fruits with vegetables are the way to go to maintain a well-balanced whole foods diet. Personally, I don't calculate exact numbers of macronutrients, and my usual meal consists of 1 part protein, 1 part carbs, and 2 parts veggies. Sure thing, you can alter this depending on your goals.

In fact, preparing food a couple of times per week can be pleasing and even entertaining which is opposite to cooking every single night. Meal prep involves planning the meals ahead of time, shopping, batch cooking and then stocking your fridge with various healthy meals, including snacks. Later in this book, we will anatomize each and every step of this amazing food prep process. And right now, we are going to focus on meal prep benefits.

Eat healthy, live longer!

Time savings

Meal prep gives you more time in the evenings to relax, work out, or do whatever you want. You have options other than rushing home to cook, and it is possible due to the cooking in bulk. Also, having things ready to go helps you save time worrying about food and ordering food during the work week. Imagine only on Sunday night you go to sleep knowing that you are set for the next few days or an entire week. In fact, food prep does not have to be an entire week; it works for you according to your schedule.

Money Saving

Meal prep helps you save your money by budgeting your grocery shopping and by not eating out. Well, we all know that dining out is expensive. Naturally, you save a significant amount of money, preparing most of your meals at home.

Batch cooking allows you to purchase more discounted bulk ingredients. As a result, you will save your money. Even more, you can base your week meal plan on what is on sale. In this case, you should plan your recipes only after grocery shopping. Eventually, you will buy fresh foods and spend less money on food. And your menu is variable enough because sales change every week. Just think about it.

Also, food prep helps to reduce the amount of food waste. Just because you plan your meals ahead, you are significantly less likely to throw out food than other people.

Food variety

When you prepare a bunch food in advance, you will have a lot of the same food, which can get a little monotonous. By focusing on cooking ingredients rather than meals, you can avoid getting bored at consuming the same thing every day. Use your ingredients in different combinations to get an assortment of go-to recipes that you can rotate throughout the week.

It's a good practice to try at least one new recipe each week. Change up different cultures, spices, and flavors to reduce food fatigue and keep it fresh. Most people follow the same routine and eat the same meals every day for years without even realizing it. Meal prep will open the fun world of food to you!

Healthier eating

Food prep helps you to get control over both the ingredients and your personal portion size. When you fueled your body with the healthiest whole foods you can possibly find, you want to work out much more.

You should not make any food choices when you're in a rush, hungry or just feeling lazy. Having your healthy meals at the ready means, you're far less tempted to eat fast-food, sweets and junk. Instead of relying on your willpower, which in most cases will fail you, meal prep allows us to plan healthy food ahead of time.

Portion control

It is a well-known fact that control of your portion sizes is the key to weight loss. But eating out and your portion control do not mix well at all. Restaurants just sell the same portion size of their dishes to every client. And meal prepping provides you with instant portion control.

To figure out your optimal portion size, make notes of how you feel after the meal and what sizes worked best for you. You should feel satisfied enough without putting yourself in a food coma. Buy the food containers of appropriate size, and you will be less likely to overeat. In the next chapter, we will consider your food containers in more detail.

And of course, if you want to lose weight, use portion sizes a bit smaller than you'd usually have and eat more non-starchy vegetables.

Consistency

Meal prepping makes consistency a lot easier since you can answer the question "What's for dinner tonight?" without any stress. You simply do not have to worry about it because it is already done. It is consistency at its finest, isn't it?

You don't have to cook thirty meals in one day to feel the benefits of food prep. If you try to prepare too much too soon, you may end up feeling overwhelmed and wasting your food. Start small and triple your favorite whole foods recipe so you can have it several times throughout the week. Your success positively will motivate you to keep going. When you see your bank account and your body change, you will naturally start to enjoy meal prep even more. It's one of the healthiest habits you can develop.

Food Prep Containers

Obviously, you need some meal prep containers, if you want your food transfer to be easy. As you already know, the size matters. I mean you should found your perfect portion size and stick to it in order to avoid feeling unsatisfied or binge eating. Eating the right portions is an equally crucial thing for losing, maintaining or gaining weight. Feel free to experiment with container sizes before purchasing a set so you can figure out your proper meal portion size.

High-quality containers last a long time; they are durable, airtight, fridge friendly, BPA free, microwave and dishwasher safe. If you are serious about food prep, investing in a few superior containers will save your money and simplify the process significantly.

Food prep containers with dividers are helpful for portioning out your protein, carbohydrates, and vegetables. And if you didn't want certain foods to touch, this option is for you too.

Small sized containers are ideal to keep snacks because you can take it in your handbag when you are on the go. And glass jars could be used for storing oats, muesli, salads, desserts, smoothies, and juices.

The amount of containers you need depends on how many meals you are going to prep per week. For entire work week, you should have, at very least, five containers for lunch and five containers for dinner. And add two extra just in case.

Failing to plan is a planning to fail!

Naturally, when it comes to meal prep, planning is the key factor. Meal planning allows you to make all healthy decisions for the week in one sitting. So in the middle of the work week, you can focus on your tasks thoroughly since you don't have to worry about being healthy. At the same time, it's not a simple and easy thing to get right the first time. But don't worry about it – you will do better next time.

For the first month, you should work your food prep into your routine. So it is clever to schedule off a block of meal prepping time so that it falls on certain days of the week. If your work timetable allows, you can do it twice a week. Anyway, you will need enough time to peel, slice, cook, and store all planned foods. In most cases, four hours are enough for prepping meals for an entire week. And it will be only two hours if you split the process to two days a week. Keep things organized, and you will do the easiest and quickest prep.

Even if you have only a few ideas for dinner, your weekly meal plan helps organize grocery shopping so you can save time and money and reduce food waste. A healthy lifestyle doesn't have to be too hard to maintain. Firstly, you have to commit to it in your mind and then plan the rest out from there. And so the next thing you need to do is make a list of your favorite healthy recipes you can depend on. Over time, you will find a core set of dishes that you know works. Versatile enough meal plan that can be used as your go-to for the months makes the food prep routine much easier.

The best thing about your **individual meal plan** is that you can incorporate your schedule and avoid prepping more meals than you need on a work week. Every week is different and this way you can take into consideration your travel, date, and days you will buy lunch at work. So take a look at your weekly schedule and **count the meals** you need to prep at home. We don't know how much food to purchase unless we look at how many meals we want to make.

	Monday	Tuesday	Wednesday	Thursday	Friday
Breakfast					
Lunch					
Snack					
Dinner					

Now decide on your dishes and write down some options for breakfast, lunch, and dinner. You should plan and cook foods you actually enjoy eating. Make sure each your meal includes a balance of vegetables, complex carbohydrates, and lean protein. Eating the same dish every single day could be boring, but you can make several different meals with a limited number of ingredients. Answer these questions in order to define your desires and possibilities:

•   What did you have last week? And what are you craving this week?

•   What vegetables and fruits are in season?

•   What meat and fish are on sale?

•   What new recipe do you want to try?

Don't choose a recipe that requires a small amount of a new for you ingredient you will never use again. Or you can try to substitute this component with a more typical product. For example, you can replace coconut milk with Greek yogurt or condensed cow milk. Contrariwise, you are going to end up throwing some of the purchased foods right in the garbage.

Before making a grocery list check your pantry, freezer, and fridge for what you need. Without this step, you are going to end up with way too much of some products. You can also correct this week's menu according to available ingredients and previously frozen meals.

Finally, make your shopping list based on the disposition of food categories in your grocery store. **Put your ingredients on the list in a particular order in which they follow each other when you walk through the store.** This way you will save your precious time and won't forget stuff on your list.

If you keep whole foods in your fridge,

You will eat whole foods!

Now it is time to go **shopping**. Don't buy on impulse and avoid soda and sugary snacks. Instead, buy fruits that are in season at the moment. Usually, they are on sale. Look for fruits and veggies that have deep colors and look heavy for their size to get the juiciest, ripest and most nutrition-packed foods.

When it comes to buying in bulk, consider which wholesale club works best for you and use it as much as possible. This way cooking in bulk saves you money. Stuff like whole grains, lentils, pasta, nuts, and seeds can last long periods of time in your pantry so don't be afraid to buy them in bulk. You can also stock your freezer with meat, fish, vegetables, fruits, and berries. By the way, some frozen foods can pack more nutrients than actually fresh. And it is a life-saving hack if sometimes you just have no time for shopping.

Canned meat, fish, beans, and tomatoes are great for some recipes. They also can sit in your pantry for months and be used when you need last-minute food prep. But please don't eat canned foods all the time!

Store ethylene-producing fruits and veggies such as tomatoes, bananas, pears, and avocados separately from ethylene-sensitive potatoes, apples, carrots, and broccoli. Also, ensure that plants are completely dry before you store them because they spoil much faster if stored wet. Remember that plant foods with higher water content like cucumbers won't store as long as something like potatoes.

The lower shelves of your fridge provide proper storage for your veggies and fruits.

On the flip side, top shelves provide the best place for cooked meals. If you are prepping on Sunday the meal that you plan to eat on Friday, put it in your freezer and defreeze it in the fridge Thursday night. So, if you plan to cook only one day during the week, you should schedule freezer-friendly dishes at the end of the week. Don't forget that some foods such as sweet potatoes and eggs do not freeze well.

Love yourself enough to eat healthy!

If you have two days for meal prep, cook the more complicated dishes on the weekend day. Cooking less complicated meals during your mid-week meal prep day helps to save energy and enthusiasm. Your oven, Crockpot or Instant Pot are just great time savers since you need just add ingredients and set it. While it is cooking one recipe, you have time to prepare another.

As a rule, meat takes a while to cook which provides you with time to get other stuff done. So, it's natural enough to cook in the following sequence: meat, carbohydrates, and vegetables. You should write down or set timers, so you will know how long everything has been preparing. Cooking several compatible ingredients gives you the flexibility to mix them together easily in a variety of ways to create quick, healthy and tasty meals. For example, baked poultry without any skin is easy enough to reheat and pair with whole grains, new sauces, and greens. You can also use it to make salad, sandwiches, or pizza.

And you can even make your own healthy minute whole grain meals. For this, cook in bulk quinoa or brown rice and cool it in your fridge. Then divide the cooked grains into meal-size containers to freeze. Now you may reheat and enjoy it anytime.

Chop and slice your veggies according to the recipe ahead of time. This way you will cut cooking time in half. Also, having chopped fruits and vegetables stimulates you to eat more salads and plant-based snacks. As a result, you will less tend to eat things like ice cream, candy bars, or doughnuts.

As lean meat, poultry is rich in protein and contains less amount of fat. Protein promotes growth and repair in your body. Also, protein helps you feel full for a more extended period of time after a meal.

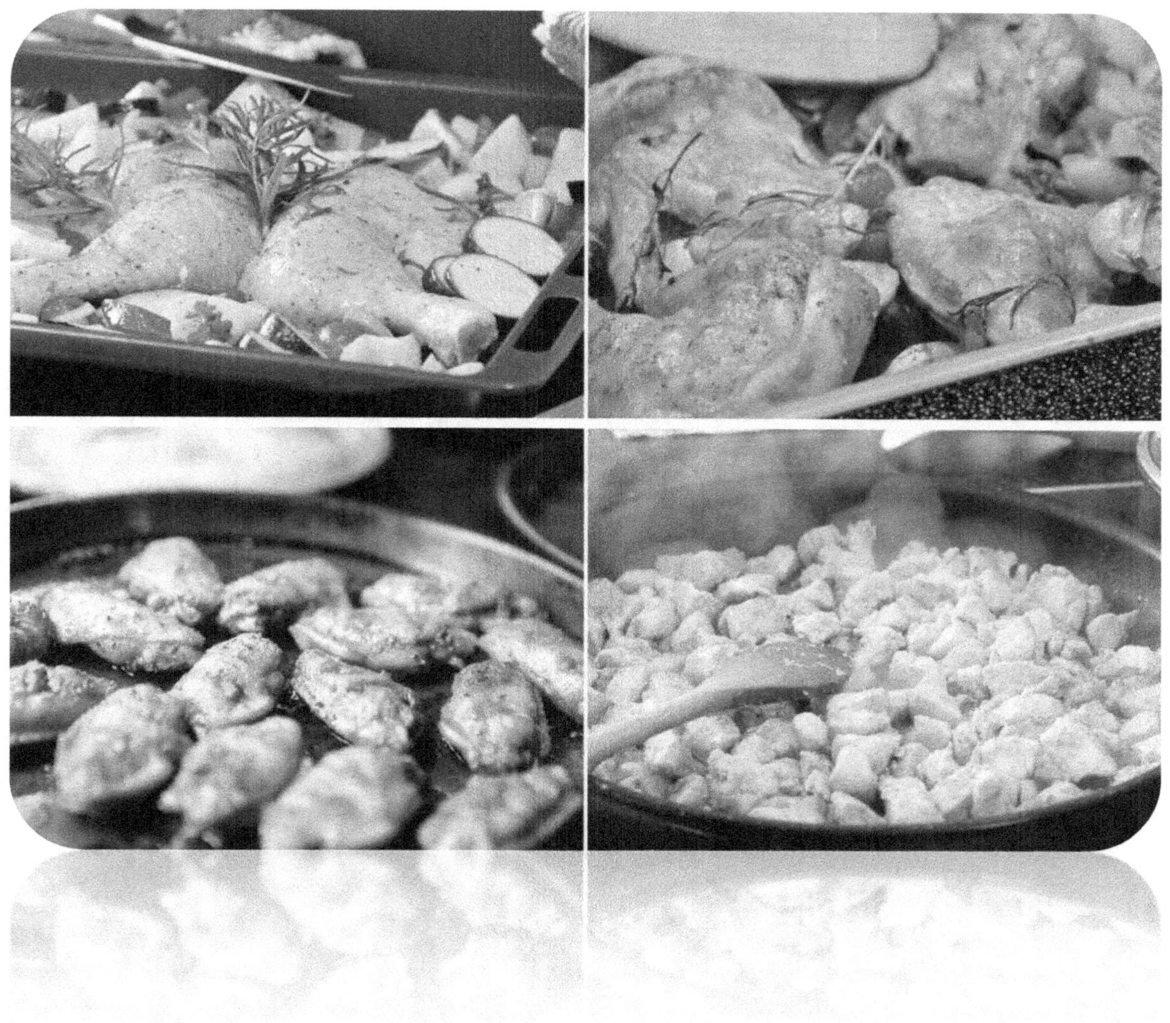

Besides protein, poultry contains several essential for our health vitamins and minerals. Poultry, being rich in B vitamins, maintain your skin health, nervous system, vision, and digestive system. Vitamin B6 and Niacin play an enormous role in preventing heart disease development.

Poultry intake aids in strong bones and teeth since it contains phosphorous and calcium. Phosphorous maintains healthy bones and teeth and improves the functioning of central nervous system, liver, and kidneys. Poultry also has selenium which is known to cut the risk of arthritis, improving metabolism, and regulating body weight.

Poultry is an excellent source of zinc which is essential for your immune system, wound healing, and hormonal balance. Notably, men should eat foods rich in zinc to regulate testosterone levels and boost the production of sperms.

Consuming poultry enhances your mood, acting as a natural anti-depressant. It contains two nutrients that are helpful for reducing stress – Vitamin B5 and Tryptophan. Tryptophan is an amino acid which increases the level of Serotonin. Also, Serotonin is one of the neurotransmitters that control depression and minimize stress.

Time: 60 mins

Number of servings: 3

Ingredients:

One pound chicken breast, cut into bite-sized pieces

One cup rice

One cup chopped lettuce

One cup feta cheese

Half cup halved olives

One chopped into wedges lemon

Juice of one lemon

One chopped red pepper

Half onion, chopped

One minced garlic clove

Two Tbsp olive oil

One tsp cumin

One tsp oregano

Salt and pepper to taste

Directions:

• In a bowl, mix together the juice of lemon, one Tbsp olive oil, garlic, oregano, salt, and pepper. Place the chicken in a plastic zip-lock bag and add the prepared marinade. Toss to coat and place in the refrigerator for forty minutes.

• Meanwhile, cook the rice according to the info on the package and add the cumin.

• In a large skillet, heat up the remaining Tbsp olive oil over medium heat. Add the marinated chicken pieces and cook for three minutes per side.

• When rice is cooked, divide it into the three containers. Add chicken, feta, olives, onions, peppers, and lettuce to each bowl. Top with lemon wedges and let your prepped meals cool down before storing in your fridge.

Time: 45 mins

Number of servings: 3

Ingredients:

One pound chicken breast, sliced

One cup brown rice

Four chopped red peppers

One chopped onion

One Tbsp olive oil

One tsp cumin

One tsp oregano

Half tsp garlic powder

Half tsp cayenne pepper

Salt and pepper to taste

Directions:

- Preheat your oven to 350°F.

- Cook the brown rice according to the info on the package.

- Line your large baking pan with foil. Then place chopped vegetables and slices of chicken on it. Pour the olive oil over veggies.

- In a small bowl, combine the garlic powder, cayenne, oregano, cumin, salt, and pepper. Cover the chicken and veggies with the prepped spice mixture and toss to coat.

•	Transfer that baking pan to the oven and cook for fifteen minutes. Meanwhile prepare three containers.

•	Remove your baking pan from the oven and transfer cooked vegetables to containers, so they're evenly divided. Then put the baking pan with the chicken back in the oven for another ten minutes.

•	When rice and chicken are cooked, divide them between containers too. Let your prepped meals cool down before storing in your fridge.

Honey-Lime Chicken with Sweet Potatoes & Asparagus

Time: 45 mins

Number of servings: 3

Ingredients:

One pound cut into smaller strips chicken breast

Three peeled and cubed sweet potatoes

Half cup honey

Juice of one lime

Two minced garlic cloves

One bunch of asparagus, ends cut off

Three Tbsp olive oil

A pinch of cinnamon

Salt and pepper to taste

Directions:

- Preheat your oven to 400°F.

- In your small bowl, mix together the honey, juice of a lime, and one of the minced garlic cloves. Stir well to combine. Place the chicken in a plastic zip-lock bag and add the prepared marinade. Toss to coat and place in the refrigerator for forty minutes.

- Line your baking pan with foil. Then place sweet potatoes on it and drizzle with olive oil. Now sprinkle cinnamon and salt over them.

•   Place this baking pan with the sweet potatoes in the middle of the oven and cook for fifteen minutes.

•   Meanwhile, heat one Tbsp olive oil in the skillet over medium heat. Add the reserved garlic and cook until fragrant. Then add asparagus, season with salt and pepper, and toss. Cook for six minutes, until asparagus, is bright green, but not too crispy. Transfer the cooked asparagus to three meal containers, so it's evenly divided.

•   Remove any remaining garlic from the skillet and add the reserved one Tbsp olive oil. Add chicken and cook over medium heat for four minutes per side.

•   Transfer the chicken and sweet potatoes to your meal containers and let them cool down before storing in your fridge.

Time: 60 mins

Number of servings: 4

Ingredients:

Four chicken breasts, skinless and boneless

One 8-oz pack of whole grain pasta

One cup shredded mozzarella cheese

One 15-oz can of crushed tomatoes

Half cup chopped onions

Quarter cup water

Four minced garlic cloves

One Tbsp sundried tomato pesto

One Tbsp olive oil

Half tsp Italian seasoning

Half tsp red pepper flakes

A pinch of dried basil

Salt and pepper to taste

Directions:

- Cook the pasta according to the info on the package.

- Season each chicken breast with salt and pepper on both sides. Heat the olive oil in your skillet over medium-high heat. Add chicken and cook for five minutes per side, until it's completely cooked through.

• Preheat your oven using broiler setting.

• Warm your skillet, add onions, and sauté for two minutes. Then add garlic and cook for just half of minute. Now add crushed tomatoes, pesto, Italian seasoning, red pepper flakes, and basil and stir well to combine.

• Bring the sauce to a simmer. Then add a quarter cup of water. Cover the lid and cook for ten minutes over low heat. Season with salt and pepper.

• Place the chicken breasts into the sauce and use a spoon to cover them with sauce. Top each chicken breast with shredded cheese. Place under the broiler for two minutes, until cheese melts.

• Finally, assemble prepared meals in your containers. Place the pasta, add some sauce and top with chicken. Let them cool down before storing in your fridge.

BBQ Chicken Drumsticks and Spaghetti Squash

Time: 100 mins

Number of servings: 4

Ingredients:

Eight chicken drumsticks

One 2-lb spaghetti squash, halved and with seeds removed

Half cup organic BBQ sauce

Two Tbsp olive oil

One tsp hot sauce

Directions:

- Preheat your oven to 400°F.

- Line your baking pan with a foil and then place halved squash cut-side down. Transfer the squash to the oven and cook for twenty minutes.

- When cooked, use a fork to pull the squash flesh and shred it into strands.

- Now coat your baking dish with oil. Put cooked spaghetti squash in the bottom of dish and top with chicken. Transfer the dish to oven and bake for thirty minutes.

- Meanwhile, in a small bowl, mix together BBQ sauce and hot sauce.

- Remove the dish from the oven and coat the chicken with spicy BBQ sauce. Then bake for another thirty minutes, coating drumsticks with sauce every ten minutes.

- Transfer the spaghetti squash to your meal containers, evenly dividing. Top with chicken and let cool down before storing in your fridge.

Buffalo Chicken Casserole

Buffalo Chicken Casserole

Time: 70 mins

Number of servings: 4

Ingredients:

One pound chicken breast, cooked and shredded

Three cups diced cauliflower

Half cup buffalo sauce

Half cup egg whites

Two chopped carrots

One diced onion

One minced garlic clove

One Tbsp olive oil

Chives for garnish

Salt and pepper to taste

Directions:

- Preheat your oven to 400°F.

- Heat the olive oil in your skillet over medium-high heat. Add onions, carrots, and garlic and sauté for three minutes, until onion is translucent.

- In a bowl, mix together chicken, cauliflower, sautéed vegetables, egg whites and buffalo sauce. Stir well to combine.

• Line your baking pan with a parchment paper and add the prepared mixture. Cover pan with the lid and bake for twenty minutes. Then remove a cover and cook for additional thirty minutes.

• Divide prepared casserole between your meal containers. Top with chives and let cool down before storing in your fridge.

Chicken Pizza

Time: 40 mins

Number of servings: 4

Ingredients:

One pound chicken breast, cut into halves lengthwise

Two cups broccoli florets, steamed

One cup diced mozzarella cheese

Half cup pizza sauce

Half cup sliced pepperoni

One Tbsp pizza seasoning

Directions:

- Preheat your oven to 375°F.

- Place chicken on a baking pan, cover with pizza sauce and top with pizza seasoning. Bake for ten minutes.

- Now Remove the baking pan from the oven and top the chicken with mozzarella cheese. Then bake for five minutes more.

- Again remove the baking dish from the oven and add pepperoni. Return to the oven and bake for an additional fifteen minutes.

- Divide prepared chicken pizza between your meal containers. Add broccoli and let cool down before storing in your fridge.

Chicken Enchilada Bowl

Time: 40 mins

Number of servings: 6

Ingredients:

Three quartered chicken breasts

One 12-oz pack of cauliflower rice

One cup enchilada sauce

Two chopped onions

Two chopped jalapeno

One 4-oz can of green chiles

Two Tbsp olive oil

Salt and pepper to taste

Directions:

• Cook the cauliflower rice according to the info on the package.

• Heat the olive oil in a skillet over medium-high heat. Add chicken and cook for three minutes per side, until lightly brown.

• Add enchilada sauce, onions, chiles, and reduce heat to simmer. Cover the lid and cook for ten minutes.

• Now remove the chicken to a platter and shred it with two forks. Return the pulled meat to the sauce and cook uncovered for additional ten minutes.

- Divide cooked rice into meal prep containers. Top with chicken, jalapenos, and sauce. Season with salt, pepper, and let cool down before storing in your fridge.

Time: 45 mins

Number of servings: 4

Ingredients:

One and a half pounds chicken breast

One 8-oz pack of button mushrooms, sliced

One cup whole wheat couscous

One cup chicken stock

Half cup sour cream

Two minced garlic cloves

One 4-oz pack of arugula

Juice of one lemon

Three Tbsp olive oil

One tsp Dijon mustard

Salt and pepper to taste

Directions:

•   Preheat your oven to 350°F and line your baking pan with parchment paper.

•   In a medium pan, bring water to a boil, add couscous and cook for ten minutes. Drain and set aside.

•   Heat two Tbsp olive oil in a skillet over medium heat. Season each chicken breast on all sides with salt and pepper and cook for three minutes per side, until lightly brown.

Transfer the chicken to a baking pan and bake for ten minutes.

•	In the same skillet, heat one Tbsp olive oil and over medium heat. Add garlic and cook for just half of minute. Then add mushrooms and sauté for three minutes, until browned.

•	Add chicken stock and simmer for three minutes, until reduced by half. Remove from heat and add sour cream and Dijon mustard. Stir well to combine and season with salt and pepper.

•	In a medium bowl, toss arugula with lemon juice and one Tbsp olive oil. Season with salt and pepper too.

•	Slice chicken and divide it into meal prep containers. Add couscous, arugula salad, and let cool down before storing in your fridge.

Time: 35 mins

Number of servings: 4

Ingredients:

One pound chicken breast, sliced into thick strips

One pound steamed green beans

One cup chopped tomatoes

Half cup plain bread crumbs

Quarter cup grated Parmesan cheese

Two minced garlic cloves

Five Tbsp olive oil

One tsp dried basil

Half tsp oregano

A pinch of rosemary

Salt and pepper to taste

Directions:

•   Preheat your oven to 400°F and line a large rimmed baking sheet with parchment paper.

•   In a shallow bowl, whisk together Parmesan, bread crumbs, basil, oregano, rosemary, salt, and pepper.

•   Pour olive oil in a separate shallow bowl and stir in garlic.

•   Dredge each chicken tender in olive oil and immediately coat with bread crumb mixture. Place them in a row along one side of your baking sheet.

•   Toss green beans with one Tbsp olive oil on the other side of baking sheet. Season with salt and pepper.

•   Place the baking sheet in the oven and bake for fifteen minutes. Then toss the green beans and cook for additional ten minutes.

•   Divide chicken and veggies into meal prep containers. Add tomatoes and let cool down before storing in your fridge.

Time: 40 mins

Number of servings: 4

Ingredients:

One and a half pounds skinless and boneless chicken breast, cubed

Four zucchini

Four minced garlic cloves

One cup sour cream

Quarter cup water

One Tbsp avocado oil

Salt and pepper to taste

Directions:

• Make noodles from zucchini using your spiralizer. Divide zoodles between your meal prep containers.

• Warm the avocado oil in a skillet over medium heat. Then add the chicken and cook for five minutes per side.

• In a saucepan, add sour cream and cook for three minutes over low heat. Then add garlic, stir, and cook for additional three minutes. Now add water, season with salt and pepper and cook for five minutes.

• Add chicken and prepared sauce in the meal prep containers and let cool down before storing in your fridge.

Time: 40 mins

Number of servings: 6

Ingredients:

One and a half pounds chicken breast

One pound asparagus, ends cut off

One cup brown rice

Two minced garlic cloves

Quarter cup oyster sauce

One Tbsp olive oil

Directions:

•   Preheat your oven to 400°F and line a baking sheet with foil. Cover with the oil.

•   Cook the brown rice according to the info on the package.

•   Meanwhile, in a small bowl, mix together oyster sauce and garlic.

•   Place chicken and asparagus on the baking sheet and drizzle with the prepared garlic mixture.

•   Put the baking sheet in the oven and bake for twenty minutes, until chicken is cooked through.

•   Divide cooked brown rice into meal prep containers. Top with chicken and asparagus, and let cool down before storing in your fridge.

Time: 45 mins

Number of servings: 8

Ingredients:

Two pounds skinless and boneless chicken breast, cut into bite-sized pieces

Two cups whole grain couscous

Three carrots, grated

Two and a half cups of light coconut milk

Two cups water

Half cup raisins

Half cup chopped cilantro

Two Tbsp curry powder

Two Tbsp flour

One Tbsp coconut oil

One tsp salt

Directions:

•   In a medium saucepan, mix together half cup coconut milk and water. Bring the mixture to a boil over medium-high heat and stir in couscous gradually. Remove from the stove, cover, and let sit for five minutes. Then open the lid and fluff it gently with a fork.

•	Place the chicken in a zip-lock plastic bag. Add curry powder, flour, and salt. Seal the bag and toss to coat.

•	Warm the coconut oil in a large skillet over medium heat. Add chicken and cook for five minutes, stirring frequently.

•	Now add carrots, raisins, and reserved two cups coconut milk. Bring the mixture to a boil and then reduce the heat to low. Simmer, stirring occasionally, for ten minutes.

•	Divide cooked couscous into meal prep containers. Add curried chicken and top with cilantro. Let cool down before storing in your fridge.

Chipotle Shredded Chicken with Cilantro Slaw

Time: 40 mins

Number of servings: 4

Ingredients:

Three cups cooked and shredded chicken breast

Four cups shredded cabbage

One chipotle pepper in adobo sauce, sliced

Two Tbsp adobo sauce (you have some in the same can with chipotle pepper)

One diced onion

One minced garlic clove

Half cup BBQ sauce

Half cup of apple cider vinegar

Two Tbsp olive oil mayonnaise

Two Tbsp chopped cilantro

One tsp olive oil

One tsp honey

Half celery seeds

Directions:

•   In a large bowl, mix together mayonnaise, quarter cup vinegar, cilantro, celery seeds, and honey. Add cabbage, stir well to combine and refrigerate for twenty minutes.

•   Warm the olive oil in your skillet over medium-high heat. Add onions and cook for five minutes. Then add garlic and cook for just one minute.

•   Now add BBQ sauce, reserved quarter cup vinegar, chipotle pepper, and adobo sauce. Cook, stirring occasionally, for eight minutes.

•   Finally, add shredded chicken and cook, stirring frequently, for five minutes.

•   Add chicken and veggies to the meal prep containers and let cool down before storing in your fridge.

Chicken Tuscan Pasta Bake

Time: 60 mins

Number of servings: 4

Ingredients:

One pound skinless and boneless chicken breast, cubed

Two cup rotini pasta, uncooked

One 8-oz pack baby bella mushrooms, sliced

Three sun-dried tomatoes, chopped

One cup shredded mozzarella

One cup milk

One cup chicken stock

Two cups chopped Tuscan kale

Two Tbsp flour

One Tbsp olive oil

Salt and pepper to taste

Directions:

- Preheat your oven to 400°F.

- In a baking pan, mix together the flour, salt, pepper, chicken stock, and milk. Then add pasta, dried tomatoes, and stir well to combine.

- Now add chicken and mushrooms, and cover the pan with a foil. Place the baking pan in the oven and bake for thirty minutes.

•   Remove the baking pan from the oven and stir everything up. Then return uncovered pan to the oven and bake for fifteen minutes more.

•   Again remove the baking pan from the oven and stir in the cheese and kale. Return to the oven and cook for another five minutes.

•   Divide cooked chicken pasta bake into meal prep containers and let cool down before storing in your fridge.

Moroccan Chicken with Veggies and Lemon Couscous

Time: 40 mins

Number of servings: 4

Ingredients:

One pound chicken breast

One cup pearl couscous

Four cups cauliflower florets

One cup chopped green beans

Half onion, chopped

Juice of half a lemon

Two Tbsp olive oil

Two Tbsp Moroccan seasoning

Salt to taste

Directions:

•   Cook the pearl couscous according to the info on the package. Stir in the lemon juice, season with salt and allow to cool.

•   Preheat your oven to 425°F.

•   Place chicken in a baking dish, sprinkle with olive oil and season with salt and Moroccan seasoning. Now put the baking dish in the oven and bake for twenty minutes, flipping once halfway. Then remove and set aside.

- Now place cauliflower florets on the separate baking sheet. Drizzle with olive oil and season with Moroccan seasoning. Put in the oven and bake for fifteen minutes.

- Remove the baking sheet with cauliflower from the oven and add green beans with onions. Then return uncovered pan to the oven and bake for ten minutes more.

- Slice the chicken into strips and divide it into meal prep containers. Add couscous, veggies, and let cool down before storing in your fridge.

Roasted Chicken and Veggies with Miso-Honey Butter

Time: 60 mins

Number of servings: 4

Ingredients:

Four chicken thighs, skin-on, and bone-in

One pound baby potatoes, halved

Sixteen Brussels sprouts, chopped in half

Half butternut squash, peeled and sliced

Four peeled and chopped carrots

Quarter cup melted butter

Two Tbsp white Miso paste

Two Tbsp olive oil

Two Tbsp honey

One tsp sesame oil

Salt and pepper to taste

Directions:

- Preheat your oven to 425°F.

- In a large bowl, add Brussels sprouts, potatoes, carrots, and butternut squash. Toss with olive oil, salt, and pepper.

- Transfer veggies to a large baking dish. Top with chicken thighs. Sprinkle chicken with oil, and season with salt and pepper. Place the baking dish in the oven and roast for fifty minutes, until chicken is golden.

•	Meanwhile, in a small bowl, mix together butter, miso, honey, sesame oil, and pepper. Stir well to combine and set aside.

•	Divide cooked chicken and veggies into meal prep containers and let cool down before storing in your fridge. Use 3-oz mini containers for miso butter.

Teriyaki Chicken with Rice and Veggies

Time: 50 mins

Number of servings: 4

Ingredients:

One pound skinless and boneless chicken breast, cut into 1-inch pieces

Two cups cooked brown rice

One cup diced baby bella mushrooms

One cup broccoli florets

Two diced bell peppers

One diced zucchini

Three chopped garlic cloves

Half cup soy sauce

Quarter cup honey

Four Tbsp olive oil

Two Tbsp vinegar

One Tbsp grated ginger

One Tbsp cornstarch

One Tbsp sesame seeds

One tsp garlic paste

One tsp chili flakes

Salt and pepper to taste

Directions:

•	Preheat your oven to 425°F and line a baking sheet with parchment paper.

•	Toss the mushrooms, broccoli, bell peppers, zucchini in olive oil and season with salt and pepper. Place all veggies on a baking sheet and roast for twenty minutes.

•	Cover chicken pieces with garlic paste and set aside for fifteen minutes.

•	Meanwhile, in a bowl, mix together ginger, garlic, honey, chili flakes, cornstarch, vinegar, and soy sauce. Add one and a half cups water and stir well to combine.

•	Heat one Tbsp olive oil in a pan over medium-high heat. Add the marinated chicken and cook for five minutes per side.

•	Add prepared sauce and bring to a boil, stirring continuously. Then reduce the heat to low and cook for three minutes.

•	Divide cooked rice, roast veggies, and teriyaki chicken into meal prep containers and sprinkle with sesame seeds. Let cool down before storing in your fridge.

Time: 60 mins

Number of servings: 6

Ingredients:

Two pounds skinless and boneless chicken breast, cut into 1-inch pieces

Four cups cooked quinoa

Two sweet potatoes, cut into matchsticks

One bunch asparagus, ends cut off

Four minced garlic cloves

Half cup pitted olives

Juice of two lemons

Five Tbsp olive oil

One Tbsp honey

Two tsp paprika

Two tsp cumin

Salt and pepper to taste

Directions:

•   Preheat your oven to 425°F and line a baking sheet with parchment paper.

•   Put chicken in a large zip-lock plastic bag. Add the honey, lemon juice, two Tbsp olive oil, garlic, paprika, cumin, salt, and pepper. Toss to coat and let chill for at least thirty minutes.

• Place the sweet potatoes on the baking sheet and toss with two Tbsp olive oil, salt, and pepper. Transfer to the oven and bake for forty minutes, flipping once halfway through cooking.

• Place the asparagus on the baking sheet and toss with the reserved one Tbsp olive oil, salt, and pepper. Transfer to the oven and cook for fifteen minutes.

• Now place the marinated chicken on the baking sheet and bake for twenty minutes.

• Divide cooked quinoa between your meal prep containers. Add chicken, sweet potatoes, asparagus, and olives. Let cool down before storing in your fridge.

Time: 40 mins

Number of servings: 4

Ingredients:

One pound skinless and boneless chicken breast, cut into 4-oz portions

Two cups cooked quinoa

One cup Greek yogurt

Two diced tomatoes

Two diced cucumber

Half onion, diced

Half cup pitted and chopped black olives

Juice of one lemon

Two Tbsp olive oil

One Tbsp red wine vinegar

One Tbsp Italian seasoning

One tsp garlic powder

Half tsp cornstarch

Half tsp onion powder

Half tsp paprika

Salt and pepper to taste

Directions:

•   Preheat your oven to 450°F and line a baking sheet with a foil.

•   In a small bowl, mix together Italian seasoning, garlic powder, cornstarch, onion powder, paprika, salt, and pepper.

•   Place the chicken on the baking sheet and coat evenly with the mix seasoning. Transfer to the oven and bake for twenty minutes.

•   Meanwhile, in a large bowl, mix together cucumber, tomatoes, onion and olives. Add one Tbsp olive oil, lemon juice, vinegar and stir well to combine.

•   Divide cooked chicken, quinoa, and Greek salad between your meal prep containers. Let cool down before storing in your fridge.

Easy Jerk Chicken

Time: 30 mins

Number of servings: 4

Ingredients:

One pound chicken breast, cut into 1-inch pieces

Two cups cooked yellow rice

One 15-oz can of black beans, drained and rinsed

Two cups diced pineapple

Half cup diced onion

Quarter cup chopped cilantro

One Tbsp olive oil

One Tbsp Jamaican Jerk Seasoning

Directions:

•   In the medium bowl, mix together pineapple, onion, and cilantro. Stir to combine and set aside.

•   Sprinkle the chicken pieces with Jamaican jerk seasoning and stir to coat.

•   Heat olive oil in a skillet over medium heat. Add chicken and cook for three minutes per side, until cooked through.

•   Divide cooked rice, black beans, chicken, and prepared pineapple salsa between your meal prep containers. Let cool down before storing in your fridge.

Time: 45 mins

Number of servings: 4

Ingredients:

One pound ground chicken

Three cups whole grain pasta

Two cups butternut squash, cubed

One 4-oz package of goat cheese

Quarter cup chopped walnuts

Two minced garlic cloves

Three Tbsp olive oil

Two Tbsp balsamic vinegar

Chopped basil for garnish

Salt and pepper to taste

Directions:

•   Preheat your oven to 400°F and line a baking sheet with a parchment paper.

•   Toss the butternut squash with two Tbsp olive oil and place on the lined baking sheet. Season with salt and pepper and bake for thirty minutes.

•   Meanwhile, cook the whole grain pasta according to the info on the package and set aside.

• Heat the remaining one Tbsp olive oil in a skillet over medium heat. Add garlic and cook for a minute. Then add ground chicken and cook for five minutes, stirring frequently.

• Reduce heat to low and add in walnuts and balsamic vinegar. Cook for three minutes and remove from the heat.

• Divide cooked pasta between meal prep containers. Top with the chicken mixture, butternut squash, goat cheese, and chopped basil. Let cool down before storing in your fridge.

Time: 30 mins

Number of servings: 4

Ingredients:

Two pounds chicken breast, cut into bite-sized pieces

Two cups broccoli florets

One cup diced tomatoes

One chopped zucchini

One chopped onion

Four minced garlic cloves

Two Tbsp olive oil

Two tsp dried basil

Two tsp marjoram

Two tsp rosemary

Two tsp thyme

One tsp paprika

Salt and pepper to taste

Directions:

•   Preheat your oven to 400°F and line a baking sheet with a foil.

•   In a small bowl, mix together basil, marjoram, rosemary, thyme, paprika, salt, and pepper.

•   Place the chicken and vegetables on the baking sheet and sprinkle with the garlic and mixed spices. Then drizzle with olive oil and transfer to the oven. Bake for twenty minutes.

•   Divide cooked chicken and veggies between meal prep containers, and let cool down before storing in your fridge.

Chicken in Peanut Lemon Sauce

Time: 65 mins

Number of servings: 4

Ingredients:

One pound chicken skinless and boneless breast

One cup brown rice

Three cups diced broccoli

Three cups diced carrots

One cup chicken stock

One cup water

Quarter cup creamy peanut butter

Two Tbsp olive oil

One Tbsp lemon zest

One Tbsp soy sauce

One Tbsp rice vinegar

One Tbsp lemon juice

Half Tbsp brown sugar

Half tsp sesame oil

Salt to taste

Directions:

- Cook the brown rice according to the info on the package, adding the salt, chicken stock and lemon zest to the cooking water.

- Preheat your oven to 425°F and line a baking sheet with parchment paper.

- Toss the broccoli and carrots with one Tbsp olive oil and place on the baking sheet.

- Place the chicken in a small baking pan and cover with one Tbsp olive oil and soy sauce.

- Transfer the chicken and veggies to the oven. Bake for twenty minutes, flipping chicken and stirring veggies once halfway through cooking.

- Meanwhile, gently heat the peanut butter in a microwave-safe dish. Then stir in lemon juice, sesame oil, rice vinegar, and brow sugar.

- Slice cooked chicken. Divide cooked brown rice between meal prep containers and top with sliced chicken and vegetables. Drizzle with prepared peanut lemon sauce and let cool down before storing in your fridge.

Time: 70 mins

Number of servings: 4

Ingredients:

One pound lean ground turkey

One cup brown rice

One 12-oz can of whole kernel corn

Two cups diced tomatoes

Quarter cup shredded mozzarella cheese

One minced onion

One minced jalapeno

Zest of one lime

Juice of half a lime

Two Tbsp olive oil

Two Tbsp taco seasoning mix

Salt to taste

Directions:

•   Cook brown rice according to the info on the package, adding the salt and lime zest to the cooking water.

•   Heat olive oil in a skillet over medium high heat. Add ground turkey and cook for ten minutes, breaking it apart with a spatula.

- In a large bowl, mix together tomatoes, jalapeno, onions, and lime juice. Season with salt and stir well to combine.

- Divide cooked brown rice into your meal prep containers. Then add cooked taco meat, prepared salsa, and corn kernels. Let cool down before storing in your fridge.

Time: 35 mins

Number of servings: 4

Ingredients:

One pound ground turkey

Four cups cauliflower rice

One cup baby spinach

Half cup chopped basil

One bunch bok choy, chopped

Two sliced bell peppers

One diced onion

Half cup coconut aminos

Three Tbsp olive oil

Two tsp minced fresh ginger

Two tsp chili paste

One tsp fish sauce

Salt and pepper to taste

Directions:

• Heat two Tbsp olive oil in a skillet over medium high heat. Add ground turkey, two Tbsp coconut aminos, one tsp chili paste, one tsp ginger, half tsp fish sauce. Stir and cook for five minutes.

- Then add chopped basil, season with salt and pepper and cook for additional five minutes. Transfer cooked turkey to a platter and set aside.

- Add one Tbsp olive oil, onions, and bell peppers in a skillet. Cook for three minutes over medium heat, until onion is translucent. Add bok choy, spinach, and cook for five minutes, until softened. Then transfer veggies to a platter and set aside.

- Pour the remaining one Tbsp olive oil in a skillet. Then add cauliflower rice, season with salt and pepper, and cook for five minutes, stirring occasionally.

- In a small saucepan, combine the remaining coconut aminos, minced ginger, chili paste, and fish sauce.

- Now divide cooked turkey, veggies, and cauliflower rice between your meal prep containers. Then top with the prepared sauce and let cool down before storing in your fridge.

Time: 45 mins

Number of servings: 4

Ingredients:

One pound ground turkey breast

Two chopped sweet potatoes

One cup chopped green onions

Two sliced tomatoes

Half of onion, sliced

Eight lettuce leaves

Two Tbsp coconut oil

One Tbsp olive oil

One tsp cumin

A pinch of cayenne pepper

Salt and pepper

Directions:

- Preheat your oven to 400°F.

- In your bowl, mix together olive oil, cayenne, salt, and pepper. Add sweet potatoes and toss to coat.

- Line your baking pan with foil. Then place sweet potatoes on it and bake for thirty minutes, flipping once halfway.

•   Meanwhile, in a large bowl, mix together ground turkey, green onions, cumin, salt, and pepper. Stir well to combine and form eight patties with your hands.

•   Heat the coconut oil in your skillet over medium-high heat. Add patties and cook for eight minutes per side.

•   Now assemble prepared meals in your containers. Place the patties on a lettuce leave, add onions and tomatoes. Then add baked sweet potatoes. Let them cool down before storing in your fridge.

Time: 70 mins

Number of servings: 8

Ingredients:

Two pounds turkey breast, skin-on and bone-in

Two bunches chopped Swiss chard

Two sliced carrots

One bunch chopped spinach

One sliced bell pepper

One sliced onion

Three minced garlic clove

Juice of half a lemon

One Tbsp olive oil

One Tbsp chopped chives

One Tbsp chopped parsley

One Tbsp chopped thyme

Salt and pepper to taste

Directions:

- Preheat your oven to 350°F.

- Disperse one sliced carrot, half of sliced onion, and two minced garlic cloves along the bottom of a baking dish.

•   In a small bowl, mix together thyme, parsley, and chives. Staff the mixture under the skin of the turkey breast. Season meat with salt and pepper.

•   Place the turkey breast in the baking dish, on top of the veggies. Then pour ¼-inch of water in the dish, place it in the oven, and bake for forty minutes.

•   Meanwhile, warm the olive oil in your skillet over medium heat. Add bell pepper and the remaining carrot, onion, garlic. Sauté for five minutes and then add a half of Swiss chard and cook until it's wilted. Repeat with remaining chard and spinach, one by one.

•   Now slice the cooked turkey and divide between your meal prep containers. Add vegetables from the skillet and let cool down before storing in your fridge.

Egg Recipes

Eggs are very popular in meal plans for both losing weight and building muscle. Due to their protein power, eggs can help to be more satisfied during weight loss process. And several studies show that egg-eaters achieve a greater reduction in waistline, compared to a control group. Moreover, an egg is a budget-friendly, easy, and versatile food.

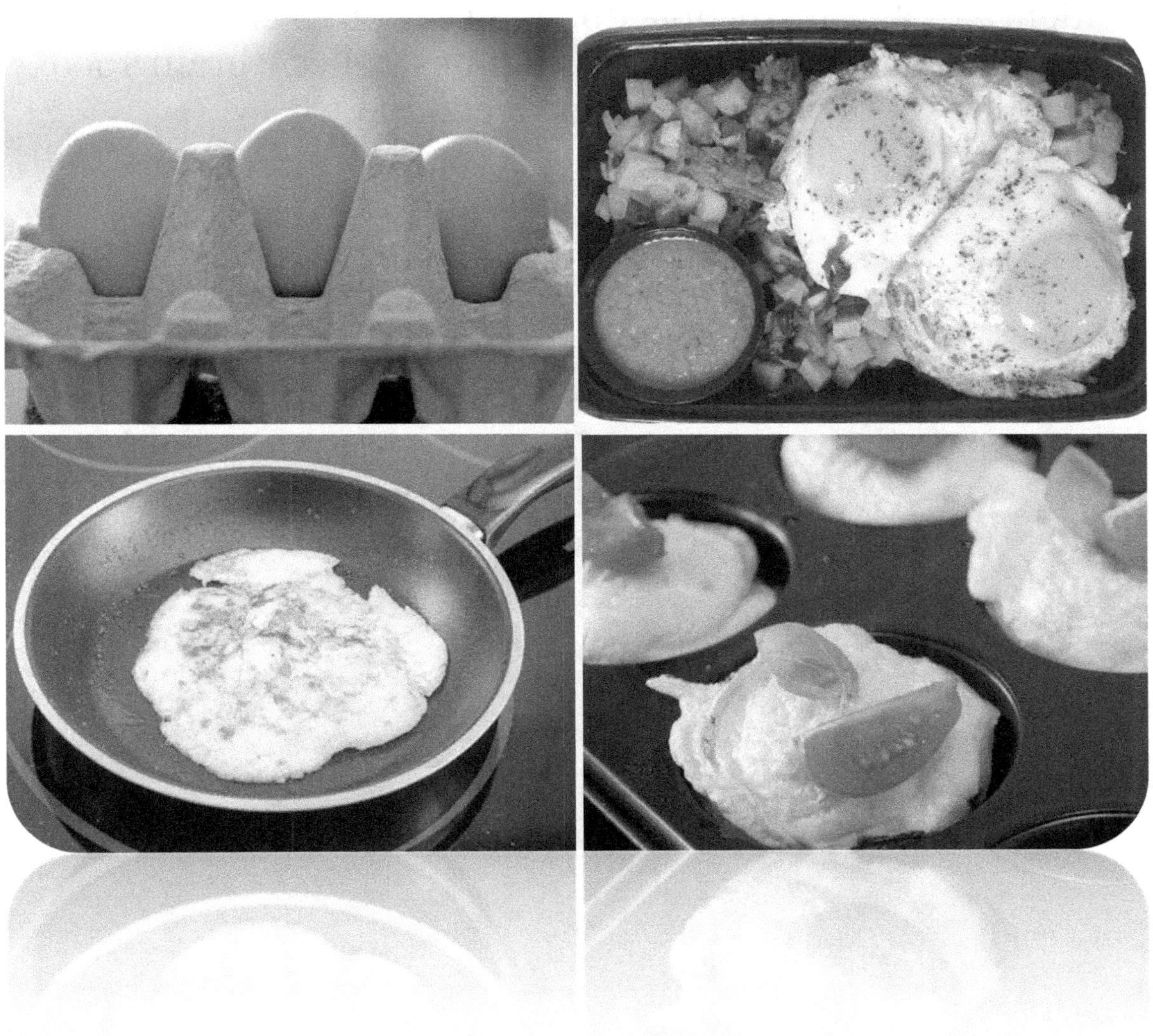

One large chicken egg has just 70 calories and provides you with 18 vitamins and minerals, and most of these essential nutrients reside in the yolk. That's why consuming whole eggs results in significantly greater muscle growth versus eating egg whites only.

One large egg satisfies about ¼ of your daily needs for choline, biotin, and selenium. Choline is a nutrient that's important for brain health, nerve function, muscle movement, and maintaining energy levels. There is some evidence that many people do not get enough choline in their diets. That's why eggs are sometimes called "brain food" - since they supply high amounts of choline.

Scrambled Eggs with Turmeric

Scrambled Eggs with Turmeric

Time: 10 mins

Number of servings: 4

Ingredients:

Eight eggs

Eight small organic sausages, cooked

Two cups broccoli florets, steamed

Quarter cup of milk

Two Tbsp olive oil

One Tbsp dried turmeric

One tsp dried parsley

Salt and pepper to taste

Directions:

•	In your large bowl, whisk together the milk, eggs, turmeric, parsley, salt, and pepper.

•	Heat the olive oil in a skillet over medium heat. Add the prepared mixture and cook for five minutes, stirring constantly.

•	Transfer the eggs to your meal containers, evenly dividing. Add sausages, steamed broccoli and let cool down before storing in your fridge.

Sausage Hash Brown Casserole

Time: 60 mins

Number of servings: 6

Ingredients:

Six eggs

Six sausages, pre-cooked

Four cups shredded potatoes

One and a half cup egg whites

One cup spinach

One Tbsp olive oil

Salt and pepper to taste

Directions:

•   Preheat your oven to 350°F.

•   In your large bowl, whisk together egg whites and eggs. Then add shredded potatoes, sausages, spinach and stir well to combine.

•   Coat your baking dish with the olive oil. Pour in the prepared mixture and bake for fifty minutes.

•   Transfer the casserole to your meal containers, evenly dividing. Let it cool down before storing in your fridge.

Veggie Egg Muffins

Time: 40 mins

Number of servings: 6

Ingredients:

Eight eggs

One chopped bell pepper

Half onion, chopped

Half zucchini, shredded

Two minced garlic cloves

Two cups chopped arugula

Quarter cup shredded Parmesan cheese

One Tbsp olive oil

Salt and pepper to taste

Directions:

•   Preheat your oven to 375°F and coat a muffin tin with cooking spray.

•   Heat the olive oil in a skillet over medium heat. Add onion, garlic, and sauté for four minutes. Then add zucchini, bell pepper, and cook for two minutes more.

•   In a large bowl, whisk together eggs, cheese, arugula, salt and pepper.

•   Now place sautéed veggies at the bottom of each muffin tin. Then fill each muffin tin evenly with prepared egg mixture. Place in the oven and bake for twenty minutes.

•   Transfer egg muffins to your meal containers and let them cool down before storing in your fridge.

Time: 40 mins

Number of servings: 8

Ingredients:

Twelve eggs

Two cups sliced bell peppers

One cup sliced organic sausage

One cup shredded cheese

Half cup heavy cream

One Tbsp olive oil

Salt and pepper to taste

Directions:

• Preheat your oven to 350°F.

• In your large bowl, whisk together eggs, heavy cream, salt, and pepper.

• Heat the olive oil in a skillet over medium heat. Then add sausage and cook for five minutes, until brown. Transfer sausage to a platter and set aside.

• Add prepared egg mixture to skillet and cook for five minutes. Then place the skillet in the oven and bake for twenty minutes.

• Remove from the oven and add sausage, peppers, and cheese. Return to the oven and broil for three minutes and then let sit for five minutes.

* Slice the cooked pizza and divide between your meal prep containers. As always, let cool down before storing in your fridge.

Time: 40 mins

Number of servings: 8

Ingredients:

Four large bell peppers, seeded and halved lengthwise

Nine eggs

Half cup black beans

Half cup cooked quinoa

Half cup boiled potatoes, chopped

Half cup shredded cheese

Half cup chopped spinach

Salt and pepper to taste

Directions:

- Preheat your oven to 400°F.

- Place the peppers on a baking sheet and cook for five minutes.

- In a large bowl, whisk together eggs, black beans, quinoa, potatoes, and spinach. Stir well to combine, and season with salt and pepper.

- Spoon the prepared egg mixture into each pepper, and top with the shredded cheese. Now place back the baking sheet in the oven and bake for twenty minutes.

- Divide cooked bell peppers between your meal prep containers, and let cool down before storing in your fridge.

Seafood provides you with high amounts of protein that tastes good. It also has low levels of saturated fat and contains vitamin E. Furthermore, fatty fish, like salmon, tuna, trout, are packed with Omega-3 fatty acids.

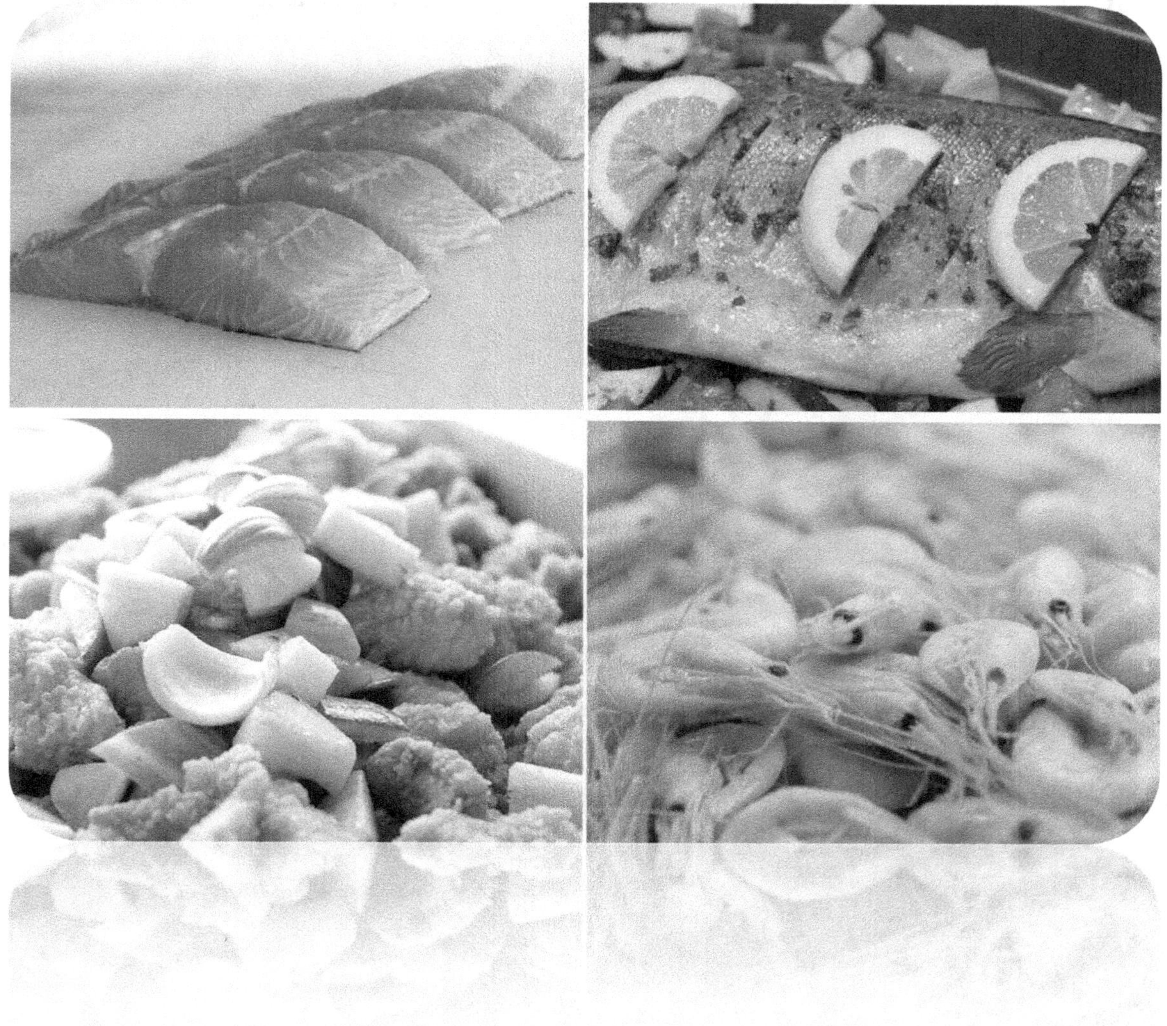

These beneficial fats can reduce the risk of heart attacks, strokes, and arrhythmias. According to statistics, regular fish consumption reduces the risk of heart attack by 40%.

Also, consuming Omega-3 can improve brain health and lower the risk of developing Alzheimer's disease. Consuming more seafood helps us have a more positive outlook on life and even has potential to treat depression.

There is a wide variety of fish and seafood to choose from. Mercury content is a serious concern with seafood. Mostly, the fish highest in healthy Omega-3 fatty acids are the lowest in mercury.

Time: 50 mins

Number of servings: 3

Ingredients:

One 12-oz pack of salmon fillets

Two sweet potatoes, peeled and cubed

Two cups broccoli florets

Two Tbsp olive oil

Two Tbsp lemon juice

One Tbsp butter, melted

Half tsp cumin powder

A pinch of garlic powder

Directions:

- Preheat your oven to 400°F

- Line the baking pan with a parchment paper and add the sweet potatoes. Drizzle with olive oil, season with cumin, salt, and pepper, and toss to coat. Put cubed sweet potatoes in the oven and set a timer for fifteen minutes.

- Meanwhile, in a small mix together melted butter, garlic powder, lemon juice, salt, and pepper. Stir well to combine.

- Line another baking pan with foil and place the salmon fillets skin-side down. Drizzle the fish with the prepared lemon-butter sauce. Now place broccoli florets on the same baking pan, drizzle them with olive oil and season with the salt and pepper.

•	When the timer on the sweet potatoes goes off, remove and flip them over. Put back in the oven along with salmon and broccoli and bake for fifteen minutes.

•	Divide the salmon, sweet potatoes, and broccoli into meal prep containers and let them cool down before storing in your fridge.

Time: 30 mins

Number of servings: 4

Ingredients:

One pound salmon fillets, cut into four portions

Two sliced bell peppers

One sliced onion

Two Tbsp olive oil

Fajita seasoning to taste

Directions:

- Preheat your oven to 400°F.

- Line the baking pan with a foil and add the salmon and vegetables. Drizzle with olive oil and season with fajita seasoning.

- Place the pan with fish and veggies in the oven and bake for twenty minutes.

- Divide cooked fish and veggies into meal prep containers and let them cool down before storing in your fridge.

Time: 30 mins (and one hour for marinating)

Number of servings: 4

Ingredients:

One pound salmon fillets

One 8-oz pack baby bella mushrooms

Four halved baby bok choy, ends cut off

One green onion, sliced

Juice of half lemon

One Tbsp sesame seeds, toasted

One Tbsp coconut aminos

One Tbsp olive oil

One tsp sesame oil

One tsp grated ginger

Salt and pepper to taste

Directions:

•   In a bowl, mix together olive oil, sesame oil, lemon juice, coconut aminos, ginger, salt, and pepper. Drizzle the salmon with the half of prepared marinade, cover, and place in your fridge for one hour.

•   Preheat your oven to 400°F and line a baking sheet with foil.

•	Place the mushrooms and bok choy on a baking sheet and drizzle with remaining marinade.

•	Place salmon skin-side down on the same baking sheet and bake for twenty minutes.

•	Divide cooked salmon and veggies between meal prep containers and top with sesame seeds and green onions. Let cool down before storing in your fridge.

Time: 40 mins

Number of servings: 4

Ingredients:

One pound salmon fillets

Two cups diced potatoes

Two cups riced cauliflower

Two cups sliced tomatoes

Two Tbsp tamarind sauce

Three Tbsp olive oil

Directions:

• Preheat your oven to 425°F and line the baking sheet with a foil.

• Toss potatoes with olive oil and place on the baking sheet. Put in the oven and bake for fifteen minutes.

• Remove the baking sheet and place salmon, skin-side down. Return in the oven and bake for an additional ten minutes.

• Meanwhile, heat one Tbsp oil in a skillet over medium heat and add riced cauliflower. Cook, stirring frequently, for three minutes. Then remove from the heat.

• Divide cooked salmon, potatoes, and cauliflower between meal prep containers and top with tamarind sauce. Let cool down before storing in your fridge.

Time: 40 mins

Number of servings: 8

Ingredients:

Two pounds salmon fillets

Juice of half lemon

Three minced garlic cloves

Three Tbsp rice vinegar

Two Tbsp chopped basil

One Tbsp soy sauce

One Tbsp honey

One Tbsp grated ginger

Two tsp sriracha sauce

Salt to taste

Directions:

• Preheat your oven to 375°F and line the baking sheet with a foil.

• Season salmon with salt and place in the center of baking sheet.

• In your small bowl, whisk together honey, lemon juice, vinegar, ginger, garlic, sriracha, and basil. Pour prepared marinade over fish and wrap tightly in the foil.

•	Bake for twenty minutes, then unwrap the foil and broil for five minutes more.

•	Divide cooked salmon between meal prep containers and let cool down before storing in your fridge.

Time: 10 mins

Number of servings: 3

Ingredients:

Two 5-oz cans of tuna in water

One cup quinoa

One cup plain Greek yogurt

Two Tbsp diced radish

Two Tbsp dried parsley

One tsp lemon juice

Half tsp fresh dill

Salt and pepper to taste

Six endive leaves

Directions:

•   In your large bowl, mix together all ingredients and stir well to combine.

•   Place endive leaves at the bottom of your meal prep containers. Then add prepared salad and store in your fridge.

Time: 40 mins

Number of servings: 4

Ingredients:

One pound sushi grade tuna, cubed

One avocado, cubed

Half mango, cubed

One cup brown rice

Two Tbsp coconut aminos

One tsp coconut vinegar

One tsp sesame oil

One tsp sesame seeds

One tsp maple syrup

A pinch of garlic powder

Directions:

• Cook brown rice according to the info on the package.

• Meanwhile, in a bowl, whisk together coconut aminos, maple syrup, vinegar, garlic powder, sesame oil and seeds. Then add tuna, gently stir, and marinate for at least ten minutes.

• Now add avocado and mix together.

• Divide cooked brown rice between meal prep containers and top with tuna poke and mango.

Time: 40 mins

Number of servings: 4

Ingredients:

Two 5-oz cans of tuna in oil, drained

One 9-oz package of egg noodles

One cup frozen green peas

One cup milk

One cup chicken stock

Half cup shredded cheddar cheese

Three Tbsp melted butter

Three Tbsp all-purpose flour

Two Tbsp breadcrumbs

Two Tbsp olive oil

Salt and pepper to taste

Directions:

• Preheat your oven to 375°F and grease your baking dish.

• In a saucepan, whisk together milk, stock, butter, and flour. Cook, stirring occasionally, for ten minutes over medium heat. Season with salt and pepper.

• Bring a pot of salted water to a boil and cook egg noodles for five minutes. Then drain them and transfer to the baking dish. Add tuna, green peas, and prepared sauce. Stir well and spread evenly in the baking dish.

•   Sprinkle shredded cheese and breadcrumbs over baking dish. Then drizzle with olive oil and transfer the casserole to the oven and bake for twenty-five minutes.

•   Slice the cooked casserole, divide it between meal prep containers, and let cool down before storing in your fridge.

Fish Taco Quinoa Bowls

Time: 30 mins

Number of servings: 6

Ingredients:

Four 6-oz tilapia fillets

Two cups cooked quinoa

One 15-oz can of black beans, drained and rinsed

One 15-oz can of corn, drained

One sliced avocado

Half cup shredded cabbage

One Tbsp olive oil

One and a half tsp paprika

One tsp garlic powder

Half tsp cumin

Half tsp salt

A pinch of ground red pepper

Directions:

•   In your small bowl, mix together the paprika, garlic powder, cumin, salt, and red pepper. Pat the fish dry and season with the prepared blend.

•   Warm the olive oil in a skillet over medium-high heat. Add tilapia and cook for three minutes per side. Then transfer fish to a platter, let cool, and cut into 1-inch pieces.

- • Divide cooked quinoa with tilapia between your meal prep containers. Then layer corn, black beans, shredded cabbage, and avocado. Let cool down before storing in your fridge.

Time: 40 mins

Number of servings: 4

Ingredients:

One pound cod fillets

One 14-oz package of pearl onions

One 8-oz package baby bella mushrooms, sliced

Two Tbsp dried parsley

Two tsp dried thyme

Salt and pepper to taste

Directions:

•   Preheat your oven to 375°F and line the baking pan with parchment paper.

•   Place the fish, mushrooms, and onions onto the baking pan. Sprinkle with parsley, thyme, salt, and pepper. Place the baking pan in the oven and bake for thirty minutes.

•   Divide cooked fish, mushrooms, and onions between your meal prep containers, and let cool down before storing in your fridge.

Chinese Style Baked Cod

Time: 50 mins

Number of servings: 4

Ingredients:

One pound cod fillet

Two cups brown rice

Two Tbsp soy sauce

One Tbsp garlic powder

One Tbsp sugar

Two tsp sesame seeds

One tsp ground ginger

Directions:

• Cook the brown rice according to the info on the package.

• Meanwhile, preheat your oven to 375°F and line the baking pan with parchment paper.

• Place the fish onto the baking pan and drizzle with soy sauce. Then sprinkle with ginger, garlic powder, sugar, and place the baking pan in the oven. Bake for twenty minutes.

• Divide cooked brown rice and cod between your meal prep containers, and let cool down before storing in your fridge.

One Pan Baked Cod with Vegetables

Time: 30 mins

Number of servings: 3

Ingredients:

Two fillets Atlantic Cod

Two cups potatoes, diced

Two cups diced tomatoes

Four Tbsp olive oil

A pinch of fresh thyme

Salt and pepper to taste

Directions:

- Preheat your oven to 400°F

- Line the baking pan with a foil and add the potatoes. Drizzle with two Tbsp olive oil, season salt, and pepper, and toss to coat. Put the pan with potatoes in the oven and set a timer for fifteen minutes.

- Remove the pan with potatoes and flip them over. Add in the cod and tomatoes. Drizzle with reserved olive oil and season with salt, pepper, and thyme. Return to the oven and bake for ten minutes.

- Divide cooked fish and veggies into meal prep containers and let them cool down before storing in your fridge.

Time: 40 mins

Number of servings: 4

Ingredients:

One pound pre-cooked shrimp, frozen

One 20-oz can of pineapple chunks, no sugar added

One Tbsp garlic powder

Half tsp black pepper

Directions:

• Preheat your oven to 375°F and line the baking pan with parchment paper.

• Place the shrimp, bell peppers, and pineapple chunks onto the baking pan. Place this baking pan in the oven and bake for thirty minutes, flipping once through the cooking.

• Divide cooked shrimp, bell peppers, and pineapples between your meal prep containers, and let cool down before storing in your fridge.

Time: 40 mins

Number of servings: 3

Ingredients:

One pound thawed frozen shrimp

Two cups chickpea pasta

One cup sliced baby bella mushrooms

Half cup Parmesan cheese, shredded

One bunch asparagus, ends cut off

One minced garlic clove

Three Tbsp butter, melted

Two Tbsp olive oil

Salt and pepper to taste

Directions:

•   Heat one Tbsp olive oil in the skillet over medium heat. Add asparagus and mushrooms and sauté for five minutes, stirring occasionally. Then transfer cooked veggies to your meal containers, evenly dividing.

•   Cook the chickpea pasta according to the info on the package.

•   Meanwhile, heat the remaining Tbsp olive oil in the skillet over medium heat. Add garlic and cook for just half of minute. Then add shrimp, season with salt and pepper, and cook for three minutes per side. Now add cooked shrimp to your meal containers in even portions.

•	Add melted butter to the cooked and drained pasta and stir well. Then add Parmesan, salt, and pepper and stir again. Finally, transfer the pasta to your meal containers, evenly dividing. Let them cool down before storing in your fridge.

Time: 20 mins

Number of servings: 4

Ingredients:

One pound shrimp, chopped

Two cups mixed chopped veggies

Two cups cauliflower rice

Two Tbsp olive oil

Two Tbsp soy sauce

Salt to taste

Directions:

•   Heat one Tbsp olive oil in your skillet over medium heat and add cauliflower rice. Cook, stirring frequently, for three minutes. In last minute of cooking add soy sauce. Then transfer to a bowl and set aside.

•   Add olive oil and increase heat to medium-high. Then add shrimp and cook for two minutes per side.

•   Now add chopped veggies, reduce heat to low, cover, and cook for six minutes. Remove from the heat and stir in cooked cauliflower rice.

•   Divide between meal prep containers and let cool down before storing in your fridge.

Time: 60 mins

Number of servings: 4

Ingredients:

One pound shrimp, peeled and deveined

Two cups cooked quinoa

One 15-oz can of black beans, drained and rinsed

One sliced avocado

Half cup chopped cilantro

Juice of one lime

One tsp soy sauce

One tsp BBQ seasoning

One tsp lemon pepper seasoning

Salt and pepper to taste

Directions:

•   Place the shrimp in a zip-lock bag. Add lime juice, soy sauce, lemon pepper, BBQ seasoning, and gently toss to coat. Seal the bag and place in your fridge for thirty minutes.

•   Meanwhile, add black beans to a saucepan, and cook for four minutes over medium-high heat. Then remove saucepan from the heat and set aside.

•   Place the marinated shrimp into a grill pan and cook for three minutes over medium heat, until bright pink.

- Divide cooked quinoa, shrimp, black beans, and sliced avocado between your meal prep containers. Let cool down before storing in your fridge.

Time: 40 mins

Number of servings: 4

Ingredients:

Four 6-oz halibut fillets, skinless

One pound peeled and chopped peaches

One cup chopped bell peppers

Half cup chopped arugula

Quarter cup green onions, sliced

Juice of two lemons

Half seeded and minced habanero pepper

One Tbsp chopped fresh oregano

Two minced garlic clove

Two Tbsp olive oil

One tsp paprika

Salt and pepper to taste

Directions:

•   In a shallow dish, whisk together one Tbsp lemon juice, one Tbsp olive oil, one garlic clove, and paprika. Add fish to the mixture, toss to coat, cover, and marinate for fifteen minutes.

•   Meanwhile, in your large bowl, mix together the peaches, bell pepper, habanero pepper, green onions, arugula, oregano, one minced garlic clove, salt, and pepper. Stir well to combine and place in the fridge.

•	Warm remaining olive oil in a skillet over medium-high heat. Remove the fish from marinade and cook for three minutes per side.

•	Divide cooked halibut and salsa into meal prep containers, and let cool down before storing in your fridge.

Time: 30 mins

Number of servings: 4

Ingredients:

Four 6-oz trout fillets

Two cups diced tomatoes

Quarter cup chopped pancetta

Quarter cup chopped fresh basil

One minced garlic clove

One Tbsp olive oil

Four lemon wedges

Salt and pepper to taste

Directions:

•   Add pancetta in a medium skillet and cook for four minutes. Then add tomatoes, garlic, salt, pepper and cook for three minutes. Remove your skillet from the heat and stir in chopped basil.

•   Warm olive oil in a large skillet over medium-high heat. Season trout with salt and pepper, and cook for two minutes per side.

•   Divide cooked trout between your meal prep containers. Add tomato mixture and top with lemon wedges. Let cool down before storing in your fridge.

Time: 20 mins

Number of servings: 4

Ingredients:

Four 6-oz tilapia fillets

Three cups basmati rice

One cup chopped bell pepper

One cup chopped green onions

Two minced garlic cloves

One 14-oz can of light coconut milk

Two Tbsp chopped cilantro

One Tbsp brown sugar

One Tbsp soy sauce

One Tbsp olive oil

Two tsp minced ginger

Two tsp red curry paste

One tsp curry powder

One tsp toasted sesame oil

Half tsp ground cumin

Salt to taste

Four lime wedges

Directions:

•   Preheat your broiler and coat a baking sheet with cooking spray.

•   Warm olive oil in a skillet over medium heat. Add ginger, garlic and cook for one minute. Then add onions and pepper and cook for another one minute. Now stir in cumin, curry powder, curry paste, and cook for one minute more.

•   Add coconut milk, soy sauce, brown sugar, and bring the mixture to a simmer. Then remove from heat, add cilantro and stir well to combine.

•   Season the fish with salt and place on the baking sheet. Broil for seven minutes, until tilapia flakes easily when tested.

•   Divide cooked fish between your meal prep containers. Add prepared coconut-curry sauce and top with lime wedges. Let cool down before storing in your fridge.

Time: 60 mins

Number of servings: 4

Ingredients:

One pound tilapia fillets, cut into six pieces

One cup breadcrumbs

Two minced garlic cloves

Two Tbsp melted butter

Salt and pepper to taste

Lemon wedges for garnish

Directions:

• Preheat your oven to 400°F and line the baking pan with parchment paper.

• In a small bowl, mix together breadcrumbs, garlic, butter, salt, and pepper. Coat the fish pieces with the prepared mixture evenly.

• Place tilapia on the baking sheet and bake for twenty minutes, until golden brown.

• Divide cooked fish between your meal prep containers. Add a side dish and vegetables of choice, and let cool down before storing in your fridge.

Red meat contains huge amounts of protein, B vitamins, vitamin D, selenium, and zinc. And half of the fats found in beef are heart-healthy monounsaturated fats. However, conventional beef has a different saturated fat profile than grass fed beef.

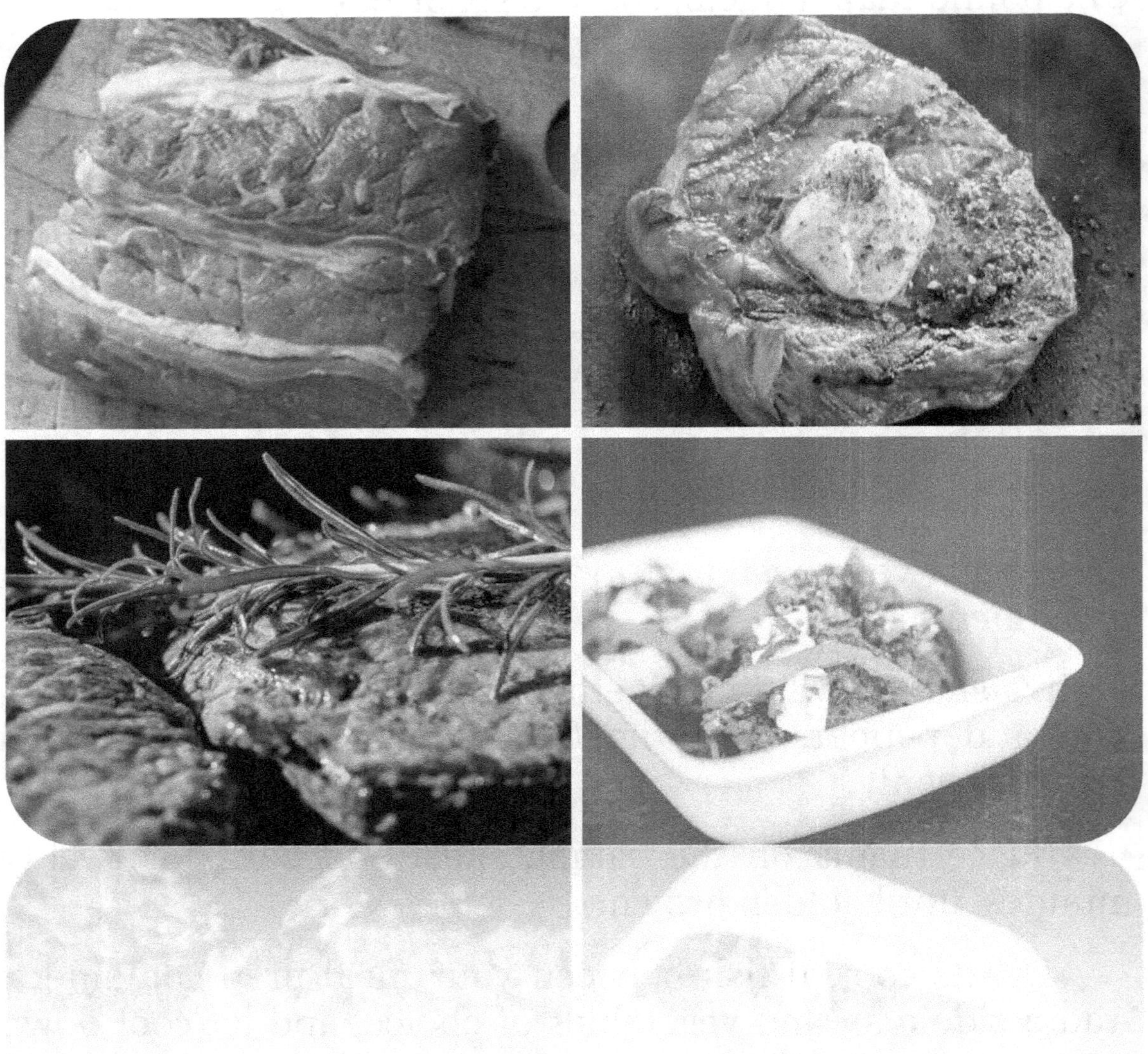

There is some evidence that many people are deficient in iron. Beef contains heme-iron - the more bio-available form of iron, which works much more efficiently than iron from veggies. Moreover, red meat has the highest rate of iron over other usually consumed meats such as poultry and pork.

Still, it is essential to limit the amount of beef you are consuming. Consider swapping some of your animal-based proteins for plant-based alternatives. Plan a couple of 'meatless' days each week.

Time: 60 mins

Number of servings: 6

Ingredients:

Two and a half pounds eye round roast

One pound Brussels sprouts, halved

Two chopped potatoes

One chopped onion

Three Tbsp olive oil

One Tbsp ground chipotle chili pepper

One Tbsp paprika

One Tbsp cumin

One Tbsp brown sugar

Salt and pepper to taste

Directions:

•   Preheat your oven to 425°F and line your baking pan with parchment paper.

•   In a small bowl, mix together chipotle, paprika, brown sugar, and cumin.

•   Heat two Tbsp olive oil in a skillet over high heat. Season the meat with salt and cook for ten minutes, turning occasionally, until golden brown.

•	Transfer the roast to the baking pan and season with the prepared paprika-chipotle mixture.

•	In a large bowl, toss Brussels sprouts, onion, and potato with one Tbsp oil, salt and pepper. Then spread the veggies onto the same baking pan around the meat.

•	Place the pan in the oven and bake for twenty five minutes. Then remove the baking pan from the oven and transfer veggies to a bowl. Return the meat to the oven and bake for fifteen minutes.

•	Transfer the roast to a large platter and allow rest for ten minutes. Then slice the meat and divide into meal prep containers. Now add vegetables and let them cool down before storing in your fridge.

Time: 60 mins

Number of servings: 4

Ingredients:

One pound ground beef

One cup shredded mozzarella cheese

One cup ricotta cheese

One cup marinara sauce

Two zucchini, peeled and spiralized

Two Tbsp olive oil

Salt and pepper to taste

Directions:

- Preheat your oven to 350°F.

- Heat the olive oil in your large skillet over medium heat. Add beef and cook for ten minutes, stirring constantly with a spatula. Then add marinara sauce and cook for three minutes more. Season with salt and pepper and let sit for fifteen minutes.

- In a small casserole dish, put layers in order: beef, zucchini noodles, ricotta cheese, beef, zoodles, ricotta, mozzarella cheese. Place this casserole dish in the oven and bake for thirty minutes. Then uncover lasagna and broil for three minutes to brown the top.

- Now slice the cooked lasagna and divide into meal prep containers. Let cool down before storing in your fridge.

Time: 20 mins (and three hours for marinating)

Number of servings: 4

Ingredients:

One pound top sirloin steak, cut into 1-inch pieces

Half cup soy sauce

One third cup olive oil

Quarter cup Worcestershire sauce

Two minced garlic cloves

Two Tbsp basil

One Tbsp parsley

Salt and pepper to taste

Directions:

•   In a bowl, mix together soy sauce, olive oil, Worcestershire sauces, garlic, basil, parsley, salt, and pepper. Stir well to combine.

•   Place the meat in a zip-lock plastic bag and add prepared marinade. Toss to coat and place the bag in your fridge for at least three hours.

•   Heat a large skillet over medium-high heat. Remove beef pieces from marinade with a slotted spoon and cook for three minutes per side.

•   Divide cooked steak pieces into meal prep containers and add veggies and side dish of your choice.

Time: 20 mins

Number of servings: 4

Ingredients:

One pound ground beef

Two Tbsp parsley

One tsp onion powder

One tsp garlic powder

Salt and pepper to taste

Directions:

•	Preheat your oven to 400°F and line your baking sheet with a parchment paper.

•	In a large bowl, mix together all ingredients and stir well to combine. Divide the prepared mixture into eight parts and form each into a meatball.

•	Place meatballs on the prepped baking sheet and bake for fifteen minutes.

•	Transfer the cooked meatballs to your meal containers, evenly dividing. Let cool down before storing in your fridge. You can add spaghetti, mashed potatoes, or steamed rice as a side dish.

Beef Burgers with Vegetables

Time: 20 mins

Number of servings: 4

Ingredients:

One pound ground beef

Two cups diced Kabocha squash

Two sliced zucchini

Four tomatoes, quartered

Two Tbsp olive oil

Salt and pepper to taste

Directions:

•   Preheat your oven to 425°F and line your baking sheet with a foil.

•   Season the ground beef with salt and pepper and divide it into eight parts. Roll each part into ball and then flatten the ball into 0.5-inch thick patty.

•   In a bowl, toss your veggies with the olive oil.

•   Place burgers and veggies on the lined baking sheet. Bake for twenty minutes flipping burgers once halfway through cooking.

•   Divide cooked burgers and veggies between your meal prep containers and let cool down before storing in your fridge.

Time: 30 mins

Number of servings: 6

Ingredients:

One pound lean ground beef

One 10-oz can of tomato soup

One cup salsa

One cup sliced mushrooms

One cup sliced onions

One cup sliced carrots

One cup frozen kernel corn

Half cup cheddar cheese

Half cup water

One minced garlic clove

Two Tbsp onion flakes

Two Tbsp olive oil

Half cup water

Directions:

• Heat the olive oil in your large skillet over medium heat. Add beef and cook for ten minutes, stirring constantly with a spatula.

•	Add salsa, tomato soup, corn, water, and cook for five minutes more.

•	Now add mushrooms, carrots, onions, and cook for another five minutes.

•	Sprinkle with cheddar, garlic, and onion flakes. Stir well to combine and divide between your meal prep containers. Let cool down before storing in your fridge.

Time: 30 mins

Number of servings: 6

Ingredients:

Six 6-oz petite sirloin steaks

One and a half cup bleu cheese crumbles

Two Tbsp olive oil

Two tsp onion flakes

Two tsp kosher salt

Two tsp black pepper

One tsp garlic powder

One tsp thyme

One tsp rosemary

One tsp coriander

Directions:

•   In a small bowl, mix together onion flakes, kosher salt, black pepper, garlic powder, thyme, rosemary, and coriander. Season each steak with the prepared blend on both sides.

•   Heat the olive oil in your large skillet over high heat. Add meat and cook for four minutes on the first side.

•   Then flip steaks and top each with bleu cheese crumbles. Cook for another four minutes.

- Divide cooked steaks in your meal prep containers and let cool down before storing in your fridge.

Time: 60 mins

Number of servings: 4

Ingredients:

One pound sirloin steak, cut into bite-sized pieces

Four chopped red potatoes

Two sliced onion

Four Tbsp olive oil

Three tsp garlic powder

Salt and pepper to taste

Directions:

- Preheat your oven to 350°F.

- In a large bowl, mix together meat, potatoes, and onion. Add olive oil and toss to coat.

- Transfer the meat-potatoes mixture to a baking dish and bake for forty five minutes.

- Divide cooked beef with onion and potatoes between your meal prep containers and let cool down before storing in your fridge.

Time: 40 mins

Number of servings: 4

Ingredients:

One pound lean ground beef

One cup brown rice

Four boiled eggs, peeled and halved

Four cups chopped spinach

Two sliced green onions

Two minced garlic cloves

Three Tbsp olive oil

Quarter cup brown sugar

Quarter cup soy sauce

One Tbsp grated ginger

Two tsp sesame oil

Half tsp sriracha sauce

A pinch of sesame seeds

Directions:

• Cook brown rice according to the info on the package and set aside.

• In a small bowl, whisk together soy sauce, sesame oil, ginger, and sriracha sauce.

•   Heat the olive oil in your skillet over medium-high heat. Add garlic and cook for one minute, stirring frequently. Then add ground beef and cook for seven minutes, stirring constantly with a spatula.

•   Add soy sauce, spinach, and soy sauce mixture, and cook for three minutes.

•   Divide cooked brown rice between your meal prep containers. Add eggs, ground beef mixture, and top with green onions and sesame seeds. Let cool down before storing in your fridge.

Time: 60 mins

Number of servings: 4

Ingredients:

One and a half pound lean ground beef

Eight halved and seeded bell peppers

One diced onion

Five minced garlic cloves

One 12-oz can of tomato paste

One 6-oz can of hot diced green chiles

Three Tbsp chopped cilantro

One Tbsp olive oil

One Tbsp garlic powder

Half tsp paprika

Half tsp ground red pepper

Salt and pepper to taste

Directions:

• Preheat your oven to 350°F.

• Heat olive oil in a skillet over medium high heat. Add onion and sauté for five minutes. Then add garlic and cook for just one minute.

•	Now add ground beef and cook for ten minutes, stirring constantly with a spatula.

•	Add tomato paste, green chiles, garlic powder, paprika, red pepper, salt, and pepper. Stir and cook for additional two minutes.

•	Spoon ground beef mixture into the pepper halves and place them in a baking dish. Cover with a foil and transfer in the oven.

•	Bake for twenty minutes, then uncover and cook for ten minutes more.

•	Divide stuffed bell peppers between meal prep containers and sprinkle with cilantro. Let cool down before storing in your fridge.

Pork has high protein containing, which is helpful to form and maintain your muscle and strengthen the immune. On the other hand, pork has high calories and fat content too. Thus, it's not recommended to consume the pork over when you are not exercising and less moving.

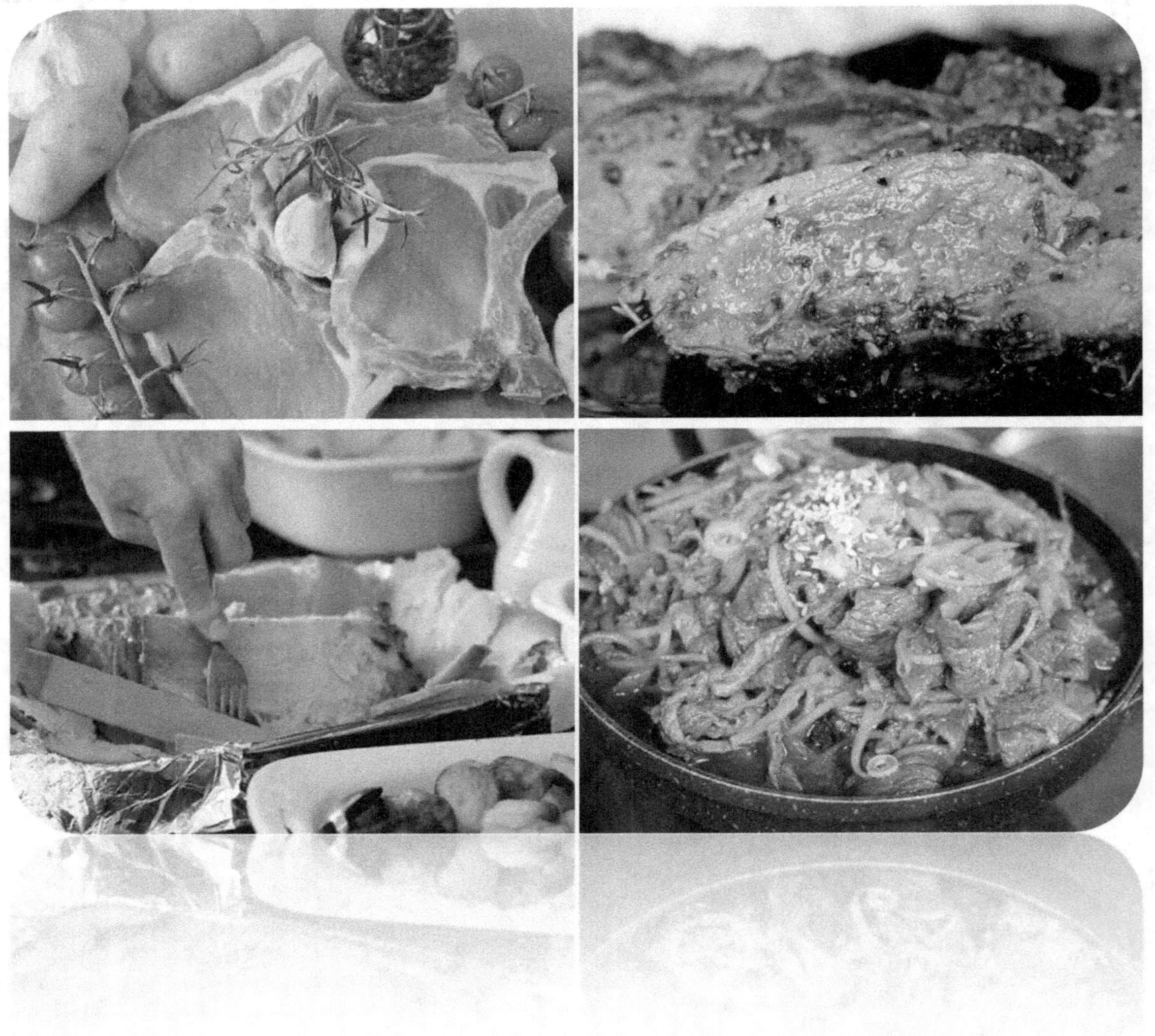

Pork is a nutrient-dense food; it's rich in Zinc, Phosphorous, Potassium, Niacin, vitamin B6, Riboflavin, and Thiamin. Thiamin is a key vitamin for protein, carb, and fat metabolism. Animal proteins are good for providing us with Thiamin, and pork is the best source among the choices.

High level of collagen is another nutritional benefit of consuming pork. Eating collagen may help to hydrate your skin, prevent joint deterioration, and minimize some signs of aging.

Time: 45 mins

Number of servings: 6

Ingredients:

Six pork chops, bone-in

Two pounds baby potatoes

Three Tbsp olive oil

One 1-oz package of ranch salad dressing and seasoning mix

One Tbsp chopped fresh parsley

One Tbsp dry oregano

One tsp ground black pepper

One tsp smoked paprika

Salt to taste

Directions:

•   Preheat your oven to 400°F and line your baking sheet with a foil.

•   In a small bowl, mix together the ranch seasoning, oregano, ground black pepper, paprika, and salt.

•   Place pork chops and potatoes on the baking sheet, cover with the olive oil and toss well. Then sprinkle with the prepared seasoning mix.

•   Place the baking sheet in the oven and bake for forty minutes.

•   Divide cooked pork chops and potatoes between your meal prep containers. Garnish with chopped parsley and let cool down before storing in your fridge.

Time: 30 mins

Number of servings: 4

Ingredients:

Four pork chops, boneless and fat trimmed

Half cup whole wheat Panko breadcrumbs

Two Tbsp Dijon mustard

One Tbsp olive oil

One Tbsp chopped parsley

One Tbsp chopped thyme

Salt and pepper to taste

Directions:

- Preheat your oven to 450°F.

- In your large bowl, mix together the breadcrumbs, parsley, thyme, salt, and pepper.

- Cover each pork chop with the mustard evenly and then dredge in the prepared dry mix.

- Heat the olive oil in your skillet over medium-high heat. Add pork and cook for two minutes per side, until golden brown.

- Now flip pork chops over and place the skillet in the oven for ten minutes.

- Divide cooked pork chops in meal prep containers. Add a side dish and veggies of choice and let cool down before storing in your fridge.

Balsamic Pork Chops with Peppers

Time: 30 mins

Number of servings: 4

Ingredients:

Four center cut pork chops

Two bell peppers, cut into strips

Three sliced garlic cloves

One Tbsp olive oil

Two tsp balsamic vinegar

Two tsp chopped fresh rosemary

Salt and pepper to taste

Directions:

•   Heat the olive oil in your skillet over medium-high heat. Season pork chops with salt and pepper, and add to the skillet. Cook for seven minutes.

•   Now reduce heat to medium and flip pork chops over. Add bell peppers, garlic, one tsp rosemary, and cook for ten minutes.

•   Drizzle the meat and peppers with balsamic vinegar and top with reserved rosemary.

•   Divide cooked pork chops in meal prep containers. Add a side dish and veggies of choice and let cool down before storing in your fridge.

Time: 50 mins (and three hours for marinating)

Number of servings: 4

Ingredients:

Two pounds pork chops, boneless

Three sweet potatoes, cubed

Two onions, sliced

Juice of two oranges

Six Tbsp molasses

Five Tbsp olive oil

Three Tbsp dried basil

Three tsp garlic powder

Three tsp cinnamon

One tsp allspice

One tsp honey

Salt and pepper to taste

Directions:

•   Place pork chops in a zip-lock plastic bag. Add molasses, juice of one orange, basil, salt, and pepper. Seal and shake to coat pork chops evenly. Marinate in your fridge for at least three hours.

- In a large bowl, mix together remaining orange juice, four Tbsp olive oil, garlic, cinnamon, allspice, honey, salt, and pepper. Then add sweet potatoes and toss to coat.

- Heat reserved one Tbsp olive oil in a skillet over medium heat. Add onions, sweet potatoes, and cook for ten minutes, stirring often.

- Add pork chops in the middle of the skillet and cook for two minutes per side. Then add marinating juices and carefully transfer the skillet in the oven, and bake for twenty minutes.

- Divide cooked pork chops with sweet potatoes in your meal prep containers, and let cool down before storing in your fridge.

Time: 50 mins

Number of servings: 8

Ingredients:

Three pounds pork cutlets, pounded ¼-inch thick

Two 15-oz cans of cannellini beans, rinsed

Four sliced bell peppers

Four sliced shallots

One cup kalamata olives, pitted and halved

One cup chopped parsley

Four Tbsp olive oil

Four Tbsp red wine vinegar

Salt and pepper to taste

Directions:

•	Season each pork cutlet with salt and pepper on both sides. Heat one Tbsp olive oil in a skillet over medium high heat. Add pork and cook for three minutes per side and then transfer to a platter. Cook all meat in three butches, adding oil every time.

•	Now heat the reserved one Tbsp olive oil in another skillet over medium high heat. Add shallots, bell peppers, salt, and pepper. Cook for five minutes, stirring occasionally.

•	Add the beans, parsley, olives, and vinegar to veggies and stir well to combine. Cook for additional two minutes.

- Divide cooked pork cutlets in your meal prep containers, and top with the vegetable mixture. Let cool down before storing in your fridge.

Time: 20 mins

Number of servings: 8

Ingredients:

Three pounds pork tenderloin, cut into medallions

Four cups cooked quinoa

Two chopped onions

Two diced apples

One cup diced mango

Half cup water

Four Tbsp Dijon mustard

Two Tbsp honey

Two Tbsp olive oil

Directions:

- In a bowl, mix together water, honey, and Dijon mustard.

- Heat olive oil in a skillet over medium heat. Add onion and sauté for two minutes.

- Add pork and cook for three minutes per side. Then add apples, mango, and Dijon mustard mixture, and cook for three minutes, until apple is tender.

- Divide cooked quinoa between your meal prep containers, and top with meat and fruits. Let cool down before storing in your fridge.

Ginger Pork Lettuce Wraps

Time: 30 mins

Number of servings: 4

Ingredients:

Two pounds lean ground pork

One 8-oz can of water chestnuts, drained and chopped

Five shredded carrots

Two diced onions

Two cups bean sprouts

One cup chopped cilantro

Half cup chopped green onions

Two minced garlic cloves

Half cup soy sauce

Quarter cup rice vinegar

Quarter cup honey

Two Tbsp Dijon mustard

Two Tbsp peanut butter

Two Tbsp sesame oil

Two Tbsp rice vinegar

Two Tbsp water

Two tsp grated ginger

Two tsp sriracha sauce

Salt and pepper to taste

Large Bibb lettuce leaves

Directions:

•   Heat a large skillet over medium high heat. Add ground pork, onion, salt, pepper and cook for ten minutes, stirring often with a spatula.

•   Add ginger, garlic and cook for just one minute. Then add quarter cup soy sauce, sesame oil, rice vinegar, peanut butter, water, and one tsp sriracha. Stir well to combine and add water chestnuts and green onion. Cook for two additional minutes.

•   In a small bowl, mix together reserved quarter cup soy sauce, one tsp sriracha sauce, honey, and Dijon mustard.

•   Spoon pork mixture into lettuce leaf. Then top with carrots, bean sprouts, and cilantro. Drizzle with prepared sauce and wrap.

•   Divide pork lettuce wraps in your meal prep containers, and let cool down before storing in your fridge.

Pork Tenderloin with Carrots and Potatoes

Time: 50 mins

Number of servings: 4

Ingredients:

One pound pork tenderloin

Half pound baby potatoes, quartered

One cup baby carrots

One Tbsp olive oil

One tsp dried thyme

Half tsp paprika

Salt and pepper to taste

Directions:

• Preheat your oven to 375°F and line your baking sheet with a foil.

• Season the tenderloin with salt and pepper on both sides. Then place meat at the center of the baking sheet.

• In a large bowl, mix together olive oil, thyme, paprika, salt, and pepper. Add carrots and potatoes, and toss to coat.

• Then transfer carrots and potatoes to the baking sheet and bake for thirty-five minutes. Remove the pork with veggies from the oven and let sit for five minutes.

• Slice cooked pork tenderloin and divide between meal prep containers. Add potatoes, carrots, and let cool down before storing in your fridge.

Time: 9 hours 40 mins

Number of servings: 12

Ingredients:

Five pounds pork shoulder

Three Tbsp paprika

Three Tbsp coarse sea salt

One Tbsp dry mustard

One Tbsp brown sugar

One Tbsp garlic powder

Directions:

•   In a small bowl, mix together paprika, coarse sea salt, dry mustard, brown sugar, garlic powder. Season the pork with prepared spice bend. Then cover and place in your fridge for at least one hour.

•   Preheat your oven to 300°F.

•   Put marinated pork in a roasting pan and roast for six hours, until it's falling apart.

•   When the meat is ready, take it out of the oven and transfer to a large platter. Allow the cooked pork to rest for ten minutes.

•   While the prepared meat is still warm, pull it with two forks. Put the shredded pork in a large container and let cool down before storing in your fridge. You can use it for prepping a wide variety of healthy meals.

Time: 50 mins

Number of servings: 4

Ingredients:

Four cups shredded pork

Two heads of broccoli, chopped

Two diced sweet potatoes

One cup BBQ sauce

Three Tbsp olive oil

Two tsp paprika

Two tsp garlic powder

One tsp onion powder

Salt and pepper to taste

Directions:

•   Preheat your oven to 400°F and line your baking sheet with a foil.

•   In a large bowl, mix together olive oil, paprika, garlic powder, onion powder, salt, and pepper. Add potatoes, broccoli, and toss to coat.

•   Then place veggies on the baking sheet and bake for forty minutes.

- Divide cooked vegetables between meal prep containers. Add shredded pork and drizzle with BBQ sauce. Let cool down before storing in your fridge.

Creamy Pulled Pork Pasta

Creamy Pulled Pork Pasta

Time: 40 mins

Number of servings: 6

Ingredients:

Four cups shredded pork

One 12-oz package spaghetti pasta

One 12-oz can of diced tomatoes

One and a half cup cheddar cheese, shredded

Half cup cream cheese

Half cup BBQ sauce

Half cup chopped green onions

One Tbsp olive oil

Directions:

•   Cook the pasta according to the info on the package and set aside.

•   Preheat your oven to 400°F.

•   Warm the olive oil in the ovenproof skillet over low heat. Add pork, tomatoes, BBQ sauce, and cream cheese. Stir and cook for one minute, until cream cheese is melty.

•   Then add cooked spaghetti, green onions, and stir until combined. Spread the pasta evenly in the skillet and top with shredded cheddar.

•   Transfer the skillet to the oven and bake for fifteen minutes. When ready, slice the pasta and divide between your meal prep containers. Let cool down before storing in your fridge.

Most veggies are naturally low in calories, so you can consume your hearty meal without worrying about counting calories. Veggies, lentils, and grains nourish beneficial bacteria in the gut, due to the fiber content. Also, soluble fiber helps you to reduce blood cholesterol. And lowering cholesterol levels reduces the risk of stroke and heart disease by keeping blood vessels clean.

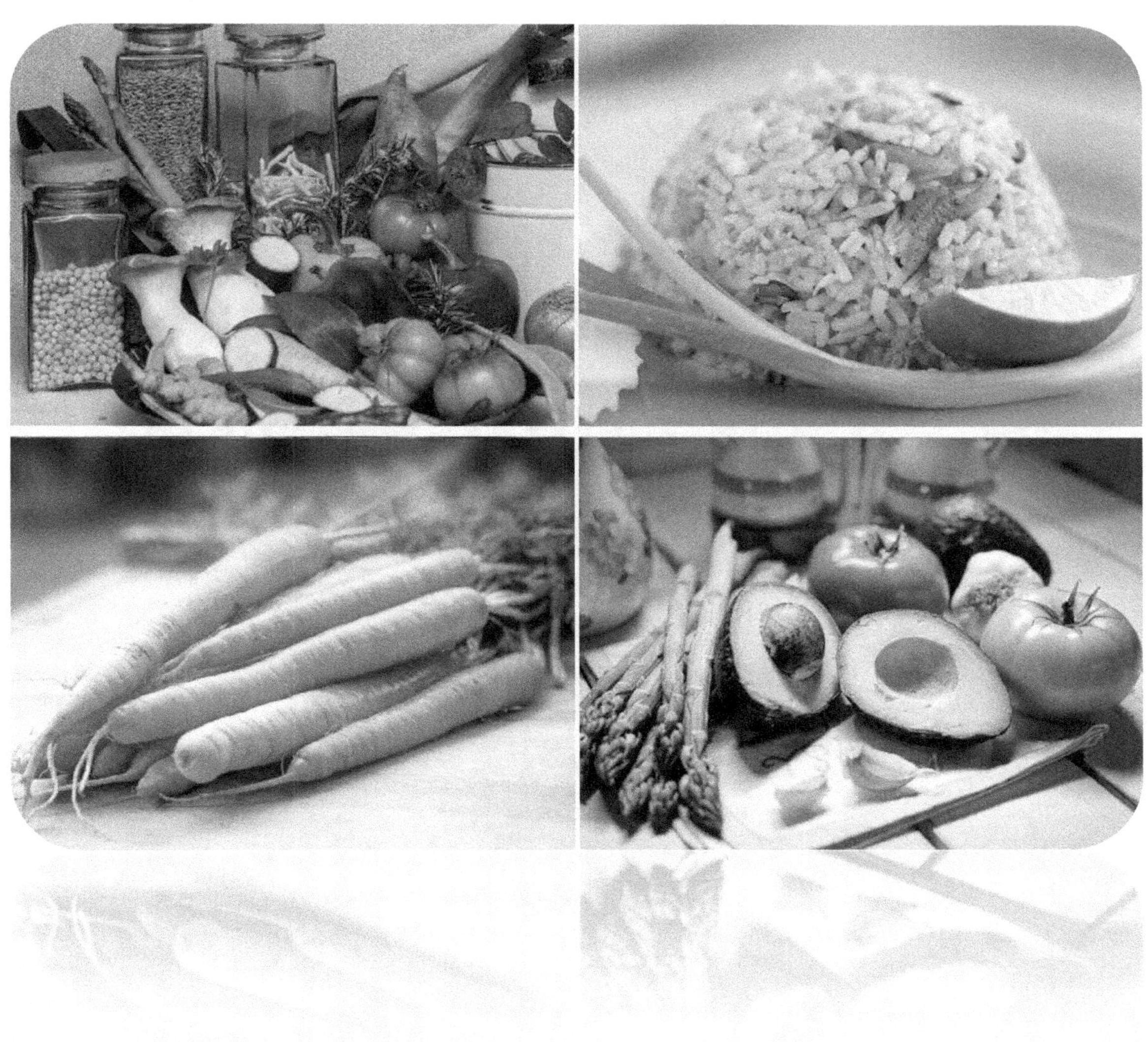

A plant-based diet is rich in vitamins C and A, potassium, folic acid and more. Although lentils, vegetables, and whole grains include all these beneficial nutrients, they are still low in fat and calories. For example, one cup of cooked lentils contains about 250 calories only and leaves you satisfied and feeling full. On the flip side, plant-based foods provide steady energy flow due to complex carbohydrates.

Time: 30 mins

Number of servings: 4

Ingredients:

Two cups cooked chickpeas

One cup quinoa

One 7-oz pack of feta

Two cups diced tomatoes

One chopped onion

Two diced cucumbers

One cup water

Half cup olive oil

Two Tbsp lemon juice

Two Tbsp honey

Two Tbsp tahini

Salt and pepper to taste

Directions:

• Cook quinoa according to the info on the package.

• Meanwhile, divide chickpeas, feta, and veggies between meal prep containers.

• In a bowl, mix together honey, lemon juice, tahini, and olive oil. Stir well to combine.

• Divide cooked quinoa in prep containers and let cool down before storing in your fridge. Store the prepared dressing in 3-oz mini containers, and add to it to bowl just before eating.

Time: 60 mins

Number of servings: 8

Ingredients:

Four cups cooked and cooled rice

Six eggs

Two cups diced green beans

Two diced onions

Two peeled and chopped carrots

One chopped bell pepper

Quarter cup soy sauce

Three Tbsp grated ginger

Two Tbsp olive oil

One Tbsp sesame oil

One Tbsp sesame seeds

Salt and pepper to taste

Directions:

•   Heat one Tbsp olive oil in a large skillet over medium heat. Beat the eggs and cook, scrambling, for five minutes, until cooked through. Then transfer to a platter.

•   Add the reserved Tbsp of olive oil, onions, ginger, and sauté for three minutes. Then add green beans, bell pepper, carrots and cook for additional five minutes.

•   Now add the sesame oil, soy sauce, and cooked rice. Stir well to combine.

•   Finally, add eggs and season with salt and pepper. Then divide in meal prep containers and top with sesame seeds. Let cool down before storing in your fridge.

Time: 30 mins

Number of servings: 4

Ingredients:

One pound firm tofu

Two cups sliced baby bella mushrooms

Two cups chopped kale

One chopped onion

One chopped bell pepper

One minced garlic clove

One Tbsp olive oil

Two tsp curry powder

One tsp turmeric

One tsp cumin

Salt and pepper to taste

Directions:

•   Heat the olive oil in your skillet over medium heat. Add garlic and cook for a minute. Then add mushrooms, onion, bell pepper and cook, stirring occasionally, for five minutes.

•   Now add tofu and break it up with a spatula. Add cumin, curry, turmeric, salt, pepper and stir well to combine. Cook, stirring occasionally, for seven minutes.

- Divide the cooked scramble into meal prep containers and top with chopped kale. Let cool down before storing in your fridge.

Time: 40 mins

Number of servings: 4

Ingredients:

One 15-oz can of black beans

One 15-oz can of pumpkin

One 15-oz can of diced tomatoes

One 15-oz can of corn

Two cups of chopped kale

One chopped onion

One chopped bell pepper

One minced garlic clove

Two cups water

Two Tbsp olive oil

One Tbsp cumin

Two tsp cinnamon

One tsp chili powder

A pinch of cayenne pepper

Salt and pepper to taste

Directions:

•	Heat the olive oil in your large pot over medium heat. Add onion, garlic, and sauté for a minute. Then add pumpkin, tomatoes with juices, and water. Stir well to combine.

•	Now add black beans, corn, bell pepper, cumin, cinnamon, chili powder, and cayenne pepper. Stir again and bring the mixture to a boil.

•	Reduce heat to low and simmer for fifteen minutes. Stir in prepped kale and season with salt and pepper. Cook for another fifteen minutes.

•	Divide cooked chili into meal prep containers and let cool down before storing in your fridge.

Time: 60 mins

Number of servings: 4

Ingredients:

One 10-oz package of whole grain pasta

Half peeled and cubed butternut squash

One 8-oz pack of baby bella mushrooms, sliced

Two minced garlic cloves

Two cups chopped kale

Two cups veggie stock

One cup milk

Two Tbsp coconut oil

Salt and pepper to taste

Directions:

•   Cook the whole grain pasta according to the info on the package and set aside.

•   Heat one Tbsp coconut oil in a large skillet over medium heat. Add butternut squash, one clove of garlic, and veggie stock. Stir well and bring to a boil. Reduce the heat to low and simmer for twenty minutes.

•   Transfer cooked squash to your blender. Add milk and blend until smooth. Season with salt and pepper.

•	In the same skillet, heat the remaining one Tbsp coconut oil over medium heat. Add mushrooms, garlic, and cook for five minutes. Then add kale and cook for another five minutes.

•	Remove from the heat and add squash and pasta to the skillet. Stir well to combine and divide between meal prep containers. Let cool down before storing in your fridge.

Chickpea and Lentil Curry

Time: 80 mins

Number of servings: 4

Ingredients:

One cup white rice

One cup rinsed and drained lentils

One cup rinsed and drained chickpeas

One 15-oz can of diced tomatoes

One 15-oz can of coconut milk

One chopped onion

One sliced lime

Two minced garlic cloves

One Tbsp coconut oil

One Tbsp garam masala

Two tsp curry powder

Two tsp cumin

One tsp minced ginger

Salt and pepper to taste

Directions:

- Cook the rice according to the info on the package and set aside.

- Heat the coconut oil in a large skillet over high heat. Add tomatoes, onion, and garlic and stir. Then reduce heat to low medium and cook for ten minutes.

- Now add lentils, chickpeas, ginger, and spices. Stir well to combine.

- Pour in coconut milk and water. Stir and bring the mixture to a boil. Then reduce heat, cover, and simmer for thirty minutes.

- Divide cooked rice into meal prep containers, add curry, and top with lime slices. Let cool down before storing in your fridge.

Time: 20 mins

Number of servings: 4

Ingredients:

Two cups cooked brown rice

One 15-oz can of black beans, drained and rinsed

One cup canned corn

One cup shredded cheddar cheese

One cup chopped kale

One chopped tomato

Juice of one lime

Two Tbsp olive oil

One tsp cumin

Salt and pepper to taste

Directions:

•   Heat the olive oil in your skillet over medium heat. Add black beans, corn, cumin, salt, and pepper. Cook for five minutes, stirring occasionally.

•   Add chopped tomatoes, stir, and cook for three minutes more. Then remove from the heat, add cheese, and set aside.

•   Divide cooked rice between your meal prep containers, add kale, and top with tomato mixture. Drizzle with the juice of lime and let cool down before storing in your fridge.

Time: 30 mins

Number of servings: 6

Ingredients:

Two cups French lentils

Two chopped cucumbers

One cup kalamata olives, pitted and halved

One cup crumbled feta cheese

Half cup chopped fresh mint

Two minced garlic cloves

Six Tbsp olive oil

Two Tbsp sherry vinegar

Two bay leaves

Two tsp whole-grain mustard

Salt to taste

Directions:

•   In a large pot, mix together French lentils, garlic, and bay leaves. Cover with water and bring to a boil over high heat. Then reduce the heat and simmer for fifteen minutes, until tender. Drain the water, discard bay leaves and garlic, and let cool down.

•   In your small bowl, whisk together sherry vinegar, mustard, and olive oil. Stir well to combine.

- In a large bowl, mix together cooked French lentils, olives, cucumbers, and mint. Pour prepared vinaigrette over salad and toss to coat.

- Divide salad between meal prep containers, and top with crumbled feta cheese. You can store this salad in your fridge for up to four days.

Lentil Shepherd's Pie with Mushrooms and Sweet Potatoes

Time: 100 mins

Number of servings: 6

Ingredients:

One cup green lentils, rinsed

One pound baby bella mushrooms, chopped

Four sweet potatoes

One cup steel-cut oats

One chopped onion

One chopped carrot

One chopped celery stalk

One minced garlic clove

Five cups water

One cup vegetable stock

Quarter cup dry red wine

One Tbsp soy sauce

One Tbsp olive oil

One Tbsp tomato paste

One tsp smoked paprika

One bay leaf

Salt and pepper to taste

Directions:

- Preheat your oven to 400°F. Place sweet potatoes on a baking sheet and bake for one hour.

- Meanwhile, in a medium saucepan, mix together lentils, oats, bay leaf, and salt. Add five cups of water and bring to a boil over high heat. Then reduce heat and simmer for twenty minutes, stirring occasionally. When ready, drain the mixture and discard the bay leaf.

- Warm the olive oil in a large pot over medium-high heat. Add mushrooms, carrot, onion, celery, garlic, and cook for ten minutes, stirring occasionally.

- Reduce heat to medium and add lentil-oat mixture, vegetable stock, wine, tomato paste, soy sauce, and paprika. Cook for five minutes. Then remove the pot from heat and season with salt and pepper.

- When sweet potatoes are ready, reduce oven temperature to 350°F. Peel sweet potatoes and mash them into a smooth paste.

- Evenly spread the lentil-mushroom mixture into a baking dish. Then top with the sweet potato mixture and smooth with a spatula. Bake for thirty minutes.

- Slice and divide cooked shepherd's pie between your meal prep containers. Let cool down before storing in your fridge.

Honey-Roasted Brussels Sprouts with Lentil-Quinoa Pilaf

Time: 50 mins

Number of servings: 6

Ingredients:

Two pounds Brussels sprouts, trimmed and halved

Two cups quinoa, rinsed

One cup green lentils, rinsed

One chopped onion

One minced garlic clove

Two cups vegetable stock

Four Tbsp olive oil

Two Tbsp honey

Two tsp cumin

Two tsp coriander

Half tsp turmeric

Half tsp cinnamon

Salt and pepper to taste

Directions:

•   Preheat your oven to 400°F. Place the sprouts on a baking sheet, drizzle with two Tbsp olive oil, and season with salt and pepper. Transfer the baking sheet in the oven and roast for thirty minutes.

•   Meanwhile, bring a large saucepan of water to a boil over high heat. Then add the lentils, reduce heat to low, and simmer for twenty five minutes. Drain and season with salt and pepper.

•   When Brussels sprouts are ready, remove from the oven and drizzle with the honey.

•   Heat the remaining two Tbsp olive oil in a large saucepan over medium heat. Add the onions, garlic, and sauté for two minutes. Then add quinoa, coriander, cinnamon, cumin, and turmeric. Stir to coat grains with the spices.

•   Now add vegetable stock, cover, and cook for twenty minutes. Then remove from the heat and let sit for five minutes. Add cooked lentils and gently fluff the mixture with a fork.

•   Divide cooked lentil-quinoa pilaf between meal prep containers. Top with the honey-roasted Brussels sprouts, and let cool down before storing in your fridge.

Time: 20 mins

Number of servings: 4

Ingredients:

Two cups boiled white beans

Four hard-boiled eggs, halved

Two chopped bell peppers

Two sliced red onions

One chopped tomato

One chopped cucumber

Two cups water

Quarter cup chopped green onions

Quarter cup chopped fresh dill

Quarter cup chopped parsley

Two Tbsp olive oil

One Tbsp lemon juice

One tsp vinegar

Salt to taste

Directions:

•   In your large bowl, mix together the beans, tomatoes, cucumbers, green peppers, green onions, dill, parsley, and olive oil.

• In your small saucepan, pour water and bring to a boil over medium-high heat. Add red onions and blanch for a minute. Then transfer them to the bowl with cold water for two minutes. Then drain and set aside.

• In a small bowl, mix together lemon juice, vinegar, and salt. Pour prepared mixture over drained red onions and let sit for five minutes.

• Transfer red onions to the bowl with salad and stir well to combine. Divide white beans salad between your meal prep containers. Top with halved eggs, and let cool down before storing in your fridge.

Time: 80 mins

Number of servings: 4

Ingredients:

Two 8-oz packages of chickpea pasta spirals

One cup brown lentils

Two shredded carrots

One sliced onion

One sliced bell pepper

Four minced garlic cloves

One 6-oz can of tomato paste

One cup halved cherry tomatoes

Half cup grated parmesan cheese

Four cups water

Four Tbsp olive oil

One Tbsp miso paste

One tsp sugar

Salt and pepper to taste

Directions:

• Cook the chickpea pasta according to the info on the package and set aside.

• Warm the olive oil in a large skillet over medium high heat. Add onions and sauté for five minutes. Then add the carrots, bell pepper, salt, sugar, and cook, stirring occasionally, for fifteen minutes, until caramelized.

• Now add the tomato paste, garlic, and cook for additional three minutes.

• Add the water, lentils, miso, and bring to a boil. Reduce the heat and cook for thirty minutes, stirring occasionally. Then add cherry tomatoes and stir well.

• Divide cooked pasta between your meal prep containers. Top with lentil Bolognese and grated parmesan. Let cool down before storing in your fridge.

Time: 30 mins

Number of servings: 4

Ingredients:

Two cups quinoa, rinsed

Two sliced bell peppers

Three sliced scallions

Two peeled and grated carrots

Two chopped cucumber

Three cups water

Half cup chopped cilantro

Half cup lime juice

Quarter cup chopped basil

Three Tbsp sugar

Three Tbsp olive oil

Two Tbsp fish sauce

One tsp salt

Half tsp crushed red pepper flakes

Directions:

• Place quinoa in a medium saucepan. Add water, salt, and bring to a boil over medium high heat. Then reduce heat to low, cover, and cook for fifteen minutes, until water is absorbed. Then transfer to a bowl and let cool down.

•	In a medium bowl, mix together lime juice, fish sauce, olive oil, sugar, and red pepper. Stir well, until sugar is dissolved.

•	In a large bowl, mix together quinoa, bell peppers, cucumbers, carrots, scallions, cilantro, and basil. Then add prepared vinaigrette and stir well to combine.

•	Divide the salad between your meal prep containers, and let cool down before storing in your fridge.

Polenta Bowls with Caramelized Onions and Kale

Time: 30 mins

Number of servings: 4

Ingredients:

One 18-oz tube of polenta, opened and cut into chunks

Four cups kale

One sliced red onion

Two cups vegetable stock

Six Tbsp olive oil

Half Tbsp garlic powder

Salt and pepper to taste

Directions:

• Place the polenta into a medium pot and turn to medium-high heat. Cook, adding a half cup of vegetable stock at a time and stirring continuously, until polenta is creamy. Then remove your pot from the heat and set aside.

• Heat three Tbsp olive oil in a skillet over medium heat. Add red onions and cook for eight minutes, stirring occasionally. Then season with salt and pepper, and set aside.

• Heat reserved three Tbsp olive oil in the same skillet. Add kale and sauté for two minutes. Then season with salt, garlic powder, and set aside.

• Divide cooked polenta between your meal prep containers. Top with kale and caramelized onions. Let cool down before storing in your fridge.

Vegetable Enchilada

Time: 50 mins

Number of servings: 4

Ingredients:

One 15-oz can of black beans, drained and rinsed

One 19-oz can of enchilada sauce

One cup corn kernels

One cup shredded cheese

Six chopped up corn tortillas

One diced summer squash

One diced zucchini

One diced bell pepper

Half onion, diced

One Tbsp olive oil

One tsp paprika

One tsp cumin

One tsp garlic powder

Salt and pepper to taste

Directions:

- Preheat your oven to 375°F.

- Warm olive oil in a skillet over medium heat. Add onion, bell pepper, summer squash, zucchini, corn kernels, and cook for seven minutes.

- Then add black beans, paprika, cumin, garlic powder, salt, and pepper. Stir well and cook for additional two minutes.

- In a medium baking dish, add half cup enchilada sauce to the bottom. Then top with two cups vegetable mixture, one cup chopped corn tortillas, half cup cheese and then another half cup enchilada sauce. Repeat all process one more time ending with a layer of shredded cheese on top.

- Place the baking dish in the oven and bake for twenty minutes, until cheese is melted.

- Remove from the oven, slice the cooked enchilada, and divide into your meal prep containers. Let cool down before storing in your fridge.

Time: 40 mins (and one hour for marinating)

Number of servings: 4

Ingredients:

One 19-oz package of extra firm tofu, drained and cut into eight parts

Three minced garlic cloves

Juice of one lemon

Juice of half orange

Half cup water

Two Tbsp soy sauce

One Tbsp grated ginger

One Tbsp sesame oil

One Tbsp rice wine vinegar

Black pepper to taste

Directions:

•   In your large bowl, mix together lemon juice, orange juice, water, soy sauce, vinegar, sesame oil, ginger, garlic, and black pepper. Stir well to combine and add tofu slices. Toss to coat, cover, and marinate in your fridge at least for one hour.

•   Preheat your oven to 190°F.

•	Place the marinated tofu in a baking dish and pour over remaining marinade. Cover the baking dish with a foil and bake for twenty minutes. Then flip up tofu and cook for additional fifteen minutes uncovered.

•	Divide cooked tofu between your meal prep containers, and let cool down before storing in your fridge.

Simple Vegetable Fried Rice

Time: 30 mins

Number of servings: 4

Ingredients:

One cup brown rice

Two cups edamame

One cup green peas

One cup corn

Two diced carrots

Two diced stalks celery

Two chopped bell peppers

One chopped onion

Half cup soy sauce

Half cup chopped green onions

Two Tbsp olive oil

One tsp grated ginger

Salt and pepper to taste

Directions:

- Cook the brown rice according to the info on the package.

- Warm the olive oil in a skillet over medium heat. Add onion, bell pepper, celery, carrot, and cook for five minutes, stirring occasionally.

- Now add rice, edamame, green peas, ginger, corn, and soy sauce. Stir well to combine and cook for another five minutes. Season with salt and pepper and remove from the heat.

- Divide cooked rice with veggies in meal prep containers, and let cool down before storing in your fridge.

Healthy Ramen Noodle Salad

Time: 20 mins

Number of servings: 4

Ingredients:

One 8-oz package of ramen noodle, cooked

Five sliced scallion stalks

Three cups shredded red cabbage

One cup grated carrot

Quarter cup chopped almonds

Quarter cup smooth peanut butter

Juice of half lime

Three Tbsp apple cider vinegar

Three Tbsp water

Two Tbsp soy sauce

Two Tbsp maple syrup

Half tsp onion powder

Half tsp garlic powder

Directions:

•   In a large bowl, mix together cooked ramen noodles, cabbage, carrots, scallions, and almonds. Stir well to combine.

•   In your smaller bowl, whisk together peanut butter, lime juice, vinegar, maple syrup, soy sauce, garlic powder, onion powder, and water.

•   Add prepared dressing to the salad and stir well to combine. Divide the salad between meal prep containers, and store them in your fridge.

Baked Sticky Sesame Cauliflower

Time: 30 mins

Number of servings: 4

Ingredients:

One chopped small head cauliflower, florets are halved

Four minced garlic cloves

Half cup soy sauce

Quarter cup honey

Quarter cup rice vinegar

Quarter cup water

One and a half Tbsp cornstarch

Two tsp sesame oil

Half tsp powdered ginger

Sesame seeds for garnish

Directions:

•   Preheat your oven to 400°F and line your baking sheet with a parchment paper.

•   Place cauliflower on the baking sheet in a single layer and bake for ten minutes.

•   Meanwhile, in a saucepan, whisk together soy sauce, honey, vinegar, garlic, sesame oil, and ginger. Warm the mixture over medium-high heat.

•   In your small bowl, whisk together cornstarch and water. Stir prepared thickener into the saucepan, when it boils. Reduce the heat to medium and cook for two minutes, stirring frequently.

•   Flip up cauliflower florets and cook for another ten minutes.

•   Divide baked cauliflower between meal prep containers, and pour prepared sauce over florets. Let cool down before storing in your fridge.

Time: 45 mins

Number of servings: 4

Ingredients:

One and a half cup farro

One 10-oz pack of lacinato kale, chopped

One 15-oz package of feta cheese, crumbled

One cup sliced artichoke hearts

One cup diced cucumber

One cup sliced bell peppers

Half red onion, sliced

Quarter cup olives, pitted and chopped

Two cups vegetable stock

Juice of two lemons

Quarter cup tahini

One bunch parsley, chopped

Directions:

•   Place farro in a large pot and pour over vegetable stock. Bring to a boil, then reduce the heat and simmer for thirty minutes. Then drain and set aside.

•   In a large bowl, mix together kale, and parsley. Stir well to combine thoroughly.

- Add farro, feta, artichoke, cucumber, bell peppers, olives, and onion. Stir well to combine.

- Divide the salad between meal prep containers, and store them in your fridge.

Time: 75 mins

Number of servings: 4

Ingredients:

One cup wild rice

One pound beets, peeled and halved

One cup toasted pecans, chopped

Two cups water

Three Tbsp olive oil

One Tbsp Dijon mustard

One Tbsp maple syrup

One Tbsp apple cider vinegar

Five sprigs fresh thyme

Salt and pepper to taste

Directions:

• Preheat your oven to 425°F

• Place beets in a large baking dish. Drizzle with one Tbsp olive oil and toss to coat. Cover the dish with foil and bake for one hour.

• Meanwhile, place the wild rice in a saucepan and add two cups water. Bring to a boil, then simmer for forty minutes.

•	In a small bowl, whisk together reserved two Tbsp olive oil, apple cider vinegar, Dijon mustard, maple syrup, salt, and pepper. Stir well to combine.

•	Cut cooked beets into bite-sized pieces and add them to the rice. Drizzle with the prepared maple-Dijon mixture and stir well to combine.

•	Divide the rice with beets between meal prep containers, and top with the pecans. Let cool down before storing in your fridge.

Actually, snacking is not necessary, if you have three well-balanced meals a day. However, in case you have that snacking habit, you should plan your snacks ahead. Meal prep helps you avoid the making decisions in the moment of hunger pangs. So, you will eat something healthy, not just sugar and empty calories.

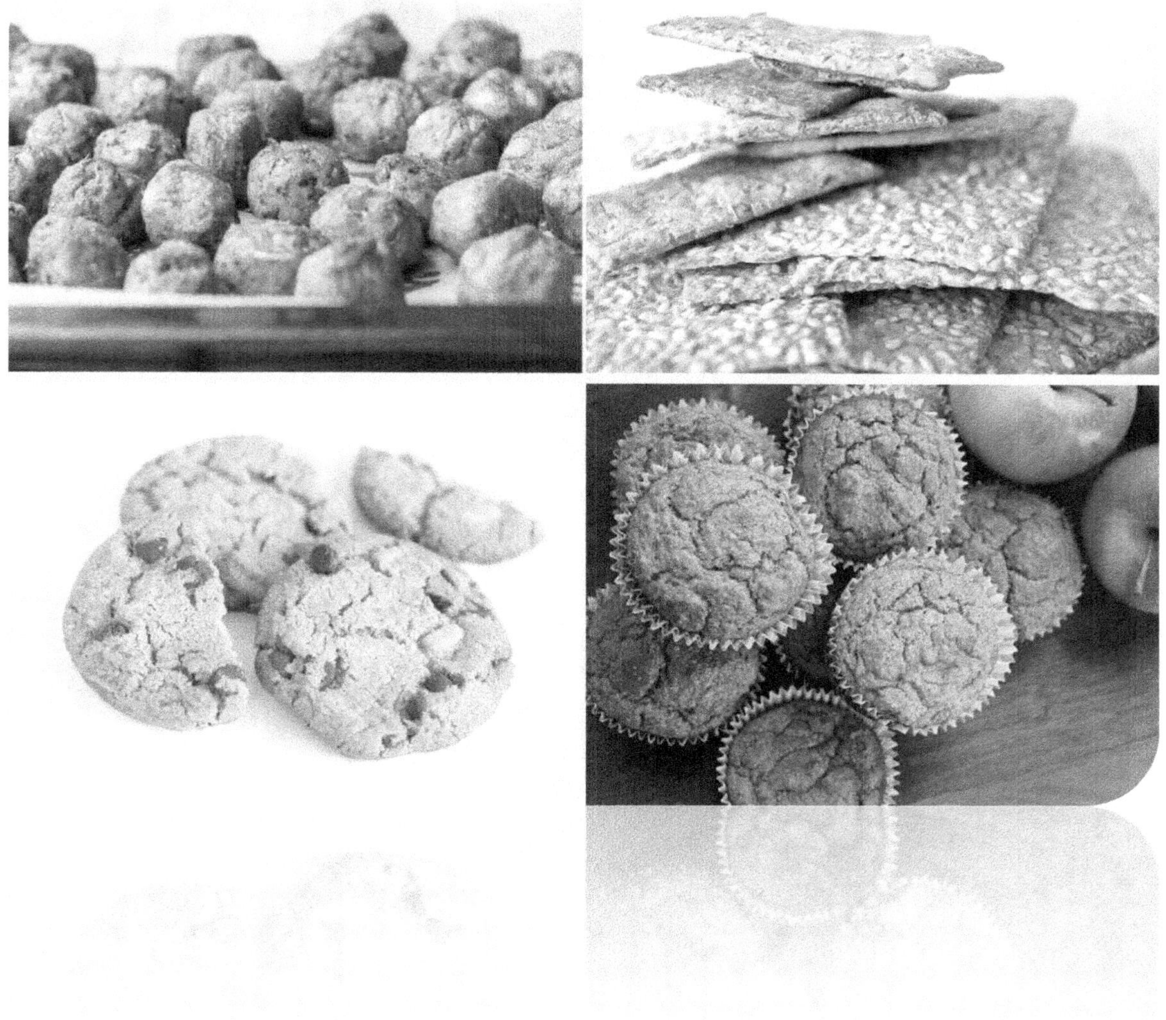

Of course, grabbing some fruit, veggie, nuts, and seeds is the easiest and quick option. It's like grabbing a candy bar, but the fruit is a nature's candy! The key to healthy snacking is planning ahead. And when you get bored with these simple options, try something new from recipes below.

Time: 30 mins

Number of servings: 8

Ingredients:

Four eggs

Half cup frozen blueberries

Half cup coconut flour

Half cup water

Quarter cup melted butter

Quarter cup Swerve Sweetener

One tsp baking powder

Half tsp salt

Half tsp vanilla extract

A pinch of cinnamon

Directions:

•   Preheat your oven to 325°F and grease a mini muffin 24-cup tin.

•   In your blender, mix together the eggs, sweetener, vanilla extract, and blend until smooth.

•   Now add melted butter, coconut flour, baking powder, salt, and cinnamon, and blend again. Let it sit for just five minutes, then add water and blend once again.

•	Divide the mixture among the muffin cups and add five blueberries to each. Transfer to the oven and bake for twenty-five minutes.

•	Divide cooked blueberries pancake bites between meal prep containers and let cool down before storing in your fridge.

Time: 80 mins

Number of servings: 12

Ingredients:

One cup of whole dates, pitted

One cup mix of dried apricots, prunes, and raisins

One cup mix of almonds, walnuts, and sunflower seeds

One Tbsp raw honey

Two tsp grated ginger

Half tsp cinnamon

Directions:

•   Place all your ingredients in your food processor and pulse for two minutes.

•   Line a large pancake pan with cellophane. Dispense the prepared mixture evenly and press until flat. Then cover and refrigerate for one hour.

•   Cut the mixture into twelve healthy energy bars. Divide in meal prep containers and store in your fridge.

Time: 35 mins

Number of servings: 12

Ingredients:

Half cup mashed bananas

Half cup unsweetened coconut flakes

Quarter cup dark chocolate chips

Two Tbsp coconut flour

Directions:

•   Preheat your oven to 355°F and line a baking sheet with a parchment paper.

•   In a bowl, mix together the mashed banana and shredded coconut. Then add coconut flour, chocolate chips, and stir well to cmbine.

•   Shape the mixture into disks and set onto the baking sheet. Bake for twenty five minutes, until golden.

•   Divide prepared cookies between meal prep containers and let cool down before storing in your fridge.

Time: 15 mins

Number of servings: 10

Ingredients:

One cup old-fashioned rolled oats

Half cup pumpkin seeds

Quarter cup peanut butter

Four pitted dates

One Tbsp chia seeds

Half Tbsp raw honey

A pinch of cinnamon

Directions:

•	Place all your ingredients in your food processor and pulse for two minutes.

•	Divide the prepared mixture into ten parts and shape each into a ball.

•	Divide prepared sweet energy bites between meal prep containers and store in your fridge.

Time: 110 mins

Number of servings: 8

Ingredients:

Half cup raw sunflower seeds

Half cup sesame seeds

Half cup whole flaxseeds

Half cup ground flaxseeds

One tsp sesame seeds

One tsp poppy seeds

One tsp onion powder

One tsp garlic powder

One cup water

Directions:

•   Place sunflower seeds in your food processor to break into smaller bits.

•   In a large bowl, mix together all seeds, onion powder, garlic powder, and water. Stir well to combine and set aside for one hour to absorb water.

•   Preheat your oven to 355°F and line a baking sheet with a parchment paper.

•   Now spread evenly prepared seed mixture on the lined baking sheet. Bake for thirty minutes, then let crackers sit in the oven for one hour.

•   Break up and divide prepared seed crackers between meal prep containers and store in your fridge.

Conclusion

Congratulations! No more looking in an open fridge trying to determine what to eat. Just grab your meal prep container and go!

Start small and prep only dinners for three days, for quick, easy, and healthy eating when you come home tired. Get good and fast at that, and then progress to adding lunches. However, you should avoid feeling overwhelmed. Don't go overboard at the start, and you will end up easily prepping breakfast, lunch, dinner, and snacks.

Add more flavor to your meals by using healthy sauces and spices. You can try a wide variety and choose your favorite. Limit consuming store-bought sauces because they contain excessive sugars, fat, sodium, and calories. Instead, whip up your own dressing or marinade with healthy ingredients like olive oil, lemon juice, grated ginger, onion, garlic, and herbs.

In order to achieve and maintain exceptional health and great shape, we need both healthy nutrition and physical activity. Naturally, your food planning should coincide with your fitness goals. Planning your workout routines and meals in the same notebook has a remarkable cross-fertilization effect!

I wish you to be healthy and happy!

Julia Schulte.